CW00603011

Measuring the quality of medical care

By
Anthony Hopkins
Director, Research Unit, Royal College of Physicians
and Consultant Neurologist, St Bartholomew's Hospital, London

1990

ROYAL COLLEGE OF PHYSICIANS OF LONDON

Royal College of Physicians
11 St Andrews Place, London NW1 4LE

© 1990 Royal College of Physicians of London
ISBN 0 900596 98 8

Typeset by Oxprint Ltd, Aristotle Lane, Oxford OX2 6TR
Printed by Antony Rowe Ltd, Bumpers Farm, Chippenham, Wiltshire SN14 6QA

Foreword

Medical audit as a method of improving the standards of patient care was the subject of a Working Party report published by the Royal College of Physicians in March 1989. Its importance has been endorsed in the National Health Service and Community Care Bill now before Parliament, and it is generally welcomed by the health profession.

The Research Unit of the Royal College of Physicians, directed by Dr Anthony Hopkins, has been set up to explore further different methods of medical audit. His monograph discusses the theory of audit and the different dimensions of the quality of medical care. There are difficulties in measuring the outcome and quality of care in medical as opposed to surgical conditions, in which audit measures can be more readily applied to a clearly defined event. Dr Hopkins discusses some ways around these difficulties, placing particular stress upon measures of the appropriateness of medical intervention, and upon the definition and measurement of the outcomes of care. He gives a number of examples of audit in practice, and describes some of the problems that others have experienced in introducing medical audit.

Measuring the quality of medical care provides a balanced account of the present status of the subject, highlights the unresolved problems, and emphasises the evolving nature of work in this field.

I believe that the information set out clearly but not dogmatically in this monograph will help all those developing their own systems for medical audit.

MARGARET TURNER-WARWICK
President, Royal College of Physicians

Acknowledgements

The Research Unit of the Royal College of Physicians is supported in part by a generous grant from the Wolfson Foundation.

I have been much aided in the understanding and development of these ideas by helpful discussions with many colleagues in the UK and the USA, to whom I am grateful.

A. HOPKINS

Contents

1 | Introduction

The 'Appropriate health care and technology programme' of the World Health Organisation has, as target 31:

> By 1990, all Member States should have built effective mechanisms for ensuring the quality of patient care.

This theme is taken up in the 1989 United Kingdom (UK) Government White Paper 'Working for Patients'[1] which requires that each health district must have in place by 1991 some system of medical audit. The White Paper defines medical audit as 'a systematic critical analysis of the quality of medical care, including the procedures used for diagnosis and treatment, the use of resources, and the resulting outcome for the patient.'

Physicians and surgeons are not used to being 'criticised'. An implicit part of their professional life is that they act at all times in the best possible faith. But criticism, as used in the arts, has a broader meaning, and is well defined by Gale:[2] 'a critic judgement is made by Experience and Prudence and Reason and Discourse' — all properties that are important in audit. Criticism has also been defined by Matthew Arnold:[3] 'a disinterested endeavour to learn and propagate the best that is known and thought in the world.' Every physician believes that he is doing his best for his patient. If he is not, the problem is an educational one.

The White Paper and subsequent Working Papers give directions for the establishment of district audit committees but do not specify their remit.[1,4] Although the Royal College of Physicians[5] and the King's Fund[6] have produced reports on medical audit, considerable confusion remains as to how health districts might usefully and promptly set about establishing audit systems. There is a need to define and understand the concepts of quality of care and to implement methods for its measurement.

This small book reviews briefly some of the work on the measurement of the quality of care, seeks to clarify some of the issues concerned, and suggests ways in which health districts may usefully undertake audit.

2 | Words we use when talking and writing about audit

First, there follows a glossary of some of the words and phrases commonly used in medical audit. By defining them we can illustrate the theoretical framework of audit within which operational methods can be initiated.

Medical audit, quality assessment and quality assurance

Medical audit is taken to imply audit of the activities of surgeons as well as physicians. *Clinical audit* embraces care given by other health professionals, eg physiotherapists. As virtually all health care involves contributions from a number of professional disciplines, the distinction is not very helpful.[6a]

The word 'audit' is unpopular with many doctors, probably because of its associations with business and accountancy — worlds which seem far removed from the care for patients. Other suggestions have been proposed such as 'systematic clinical review', but the use of the word audit in recent reports[1, 4-6] means that the term is probably here to stay. And in truth it is a perfectly adequate term. Audit is based upon *audire,* Latin for 'to hear': accounts of money spent were originally given orally.[7] The term audit in accountancy has come to mean an examination of accounts supported by written invoices for goods or services and receipts for disbursements. The simplest example of medical audit is when a physician's team is asked to support its actions by similar reference to the written record. Some writers confine medical audit to this specific task, referring to other methods of measuring quality of care as *quality assessment,* and the systems for ensuring quality as *quality assurance.*

Stone[6a] draws a distinction between ad hoc *reviews,* as opposed to continuing *audit.* He also distinguishes between an ad hoc *evaluation* of some aspect of health care, as opposed to *surveillance,* which is concerned with detecting changes in health status and potential environmental hazards over time. He suggests that we use the word *monitoring* for the more managerial counterpart of on-going data collection and analysis in the sphere of health care delivery. Finally, *appraisal* could be used for an ad hoc managerial assessment of the strengths and weaknesses of a service.

Quality of care

Brook and Kosecoff[8] define quality of care as representing

> the performance of specific activities in a manner that either increases or at least prevents the deterioration in health status that would have occurred as a function of a disease or condition. Employing this definition, quality of care consists of two components: 1. the selection of the right activity or task or contribution of activities, and 2. the performance of those activities in a manner that produces the best outcome.

Few could quarrel with this pure definition of quality, but in itself it gives insufficient meat on which to chew. A way forward is to consider the *dimensions of quality* — for example, the technical competence of the physician or surgeon, and his interpersonal skills. Once these dimensions have been defined, it is then possible to consider the methodology to be employed in measuring them.

Dimensions of quality

The generally acknowledged guru of medical audit and quality assurance is Donabedian.[9-14] As long ago as 1966, he suggested that the quality of care of patients could be audited in three dimensions — *structure, process and outcome.*

By *structure* is meant, for example, the availability of suitable buildings, equipment and numbers of adequately trained staff. If a health district has a small number of medical beds to care for acutely ill patients, it may *a priori* be suspected that the overall quality of care in that district may be less good than in a better endowed district. Although structural characteristics can readily be audited, they are unlikely to be a good guide to the quality of care. Bad care can occur in well equipped hospitals.

Process refers to the activities of medical care — the choice of investigation or operation, the use of outpatient or inpatient facilities, the number of days bed-rest specified after a surgical intervention etc. A review of hospital records can audit only the process of care and some immediate outcomes.

Outcome refers to the change in the patient's current or future health that can be attributed to a medical intervention, or other type of antecedent care. Unless the outcome after a medical intervention is an improvement in the present or future health of a patient, the activity has been meaningless, however fine the structure and however careful the process.

Measures of the process of care, such as auditing hospital records, are valid measures of quality only in so far as they relate to outcome;[10] a physician may provide excellent humane and technically successful care but write dreadful records. Equally, outcomes are only valid measures of quality to the extent that they relate to the antecedent process of care; at its simplest, patients may get better with no care at all! It is clear therefore that process and outcome measures are complementary and not rival measures of quality. However, as outcome measures other than mortality are often difficult to define (see p. 44), much audit concentrates upon process of care as a proxy for outcome. For example, if a health district achieves a high level of uptake of rubella immunisation, then a good outcome in terms of a reduction in numbers of pregnancies affected by rubella can reasonably be supposed. Two other recent examples: McCance and colleagues have shown that the development of diabetic retinopathy is clearly linked to long-term glycaemic control;[15] adherence to a treatment protocol significantly improves the survival of patients with myeloma.[16] However, process of care is not necessarily linked to outcome if only medical outcome measures are used. For example, it is very difficult to show that any treatment has any effect upon the long-term biology of multiple sclerosis, but reasonably good outcomes may be achieved by attention to alterations to the patient's home and facilities for transport, and advice about work. Attention to these aspects of care would clearly indicate a process of care of good quality.

Efficacy, effectiveness and efficiency[17]

Does treatment work? Or, more formally, do clinical interventions influence outcome?

The principal concern of clinical researchers in the last twenty years has been to measure or compare the efficacy of treatment. By randomised controlled trials it can be shown for example, that drug A is more efficacious at reducing blood pressure than drug B. *Efficacy* is defined as the ability of a medical or surgical intervention to produce the desired outcome in a defined population under ideal conditions. It must be distinguished from *effectiveness*, which is the extent to which that outcome is achieved under the usual conditions of care in 'real life', where skills and other resources are less than under the experimental conditions. For both efficacy and effectiveness, the technical competence of the providers of care is an important variable.

In an ideal world, resources would allow effectiveness to equal efficacy. However, resources are finite, and it is necessary to consider also *efficiency* — the extent to which resources are consumed by the interventions relative to their effectiveness. An efficient intervention is one which maximises the outcome(s) for given resources.

As an example of the inter-relation between these words, consider the case of coronary bypass surgery. It is *efficacious* in reducing mortality over the next five years in patients with chronic stable angina and left main-stem coronary disease.[18] In the best prospective studies, mortality is as low as 0.5%.[18] However, in general use, operative mortality is higher,[18, 19] and the five-year survival is less, so the procedure is not as *effective* as had been hoped. Large units with skilled staff can perform effective operations at lower marginal cost than those units undertaking only a few procedures each month — that is to say larger units are more *efficient.*

Appropriate care

Care that is appropriate has been well defined by workers at the RAND Corporation:[18, 20]

> Appropriate (care means) that the expected health benefit (ie increased life expectancy, relief of pain, reduction in anxiety, improved functional capacity) exceeds the expected negative consequences (ie mortality, morbidity, anxiety of anticipating the procedure, pain produced by the procedure, misleading or false diagnoses, time lost from work) by a sufficiently wide margin that the procedure is worth doing.

Inappropriate care includes both over-use and under-use of medical expertise and facilities (see Regional Variations, p. 16).

Rights to care

It is well recognised that *wants* for health care — an individual's recognition of his desire for care — are not the same as his *needs* — a call for medical interventions for deficiencies of health determined by health professionals. As King has written[21]:

> By adding 'rights' to 'wants' and 'needs', we make a difficult pair into an even more difficult trio. The right to personal health care can be considered as a group of interventions that an individual will only sometimes need, may not always want, which are not to be imposed upon him, but which must be available.

The 'right' to care will vary in different societies, but many would agree that it is more appropriate to provide in developing countries efficient and effective prevention and treatment of common infectious illnesses, and efficient and effective maternal and child health services, rather than 'high-tech' hospitals in a few urban sites.

Ethical care

Good quality medical care cannot include unethical procedures, such as the transplantation of organs sold for cash, however skilled the technical procedure, and however satisfactory the outcome.

Other dimensions of quality of care

So far we have identified ethical, effective, appropriate and efficient dimensions of quality of care. Maxwell[22] and Tarlov and colleagues[23] have also drawn attention to other aspects.

Care should be *relevant* to the needs of the community. For example, in a district in which live many black people, it would be relevant to provide sickle-cell counselling and screening services.

Care should be delivered *equitably* between different client and ethnic groups.[24, 25] As an example of inequitable care, it may be found that the chances of receiving a hip replacement are related to mode of referral or ethnic group, rather than to degree of disability and handicap. Inequitable care may also arise from professional interest in different classes of patients, so that 'interesting' patients are given priority.[26]

Care should be *accessible*, geographically, and at times that are convenient to the patient. Care should also be financially accessible, ie affordable, or provided free through national systems of taxation.

Tarlov and colleagues also consider *continuity of care* — the extent to which a patient sees the same provider(s) on successive visits, and to which a patient can identify the doctor principally responsible for his care. *Co-ordination of care* refers to the extent to which a patient's primary doctor is aware of all treatments that a patient is receiving, and communicates with other professionals concerned in his patient's care.

Care should be *socially acceptable*. It should reflect what the potential consumers want, and the way in which it is provided should satisfy their expectations. Tarlov and colleagues[23] call attention in this domain to a number of aspects of the interpersonal skills of the providers of care — notably friendliness, courtesy, respect and sensitivity, and the overall level of communication.

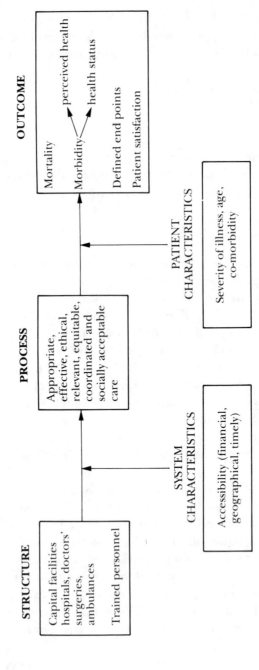

Fig. 1. *Schematic representation of some dimensions that it is necessary to consider when measuring the quality of care.*

The care should be provided in a manner that is *acceptable to its providers* — not only because the providers themselves are potential consumers of care at some time in their lives, but also because it may be presumed that a happy and involved workforce is more likely to provide care of good quality.

Finally, when considering the quality of care, it is necessary to specify the recipients of care. Are we considering care provided to a whole population — a health care system — or a sub-section of that population, for example people in a single health district? Or are we considering a well person, who receives information promoting health or undergoes some screening test, or are we considering a patient with symptoms? Measures of quality that are appropriate for one target may be inappropriate for another.

Figure 1 summarises the arguments to this point. Accessibility potentially limits the patient's interactions with structures for care; severity of illness and other patient characteristics influence the link between process and outcome.

We now consider how quality can be measured, reliably, validly and sensitively.

3 | Methods of measurement of quality of care

Methods used when attempting to measure the quality of care will now be reviewed in the order set out in Table 1.

Table 1. Examples of areas in which we should attempt to measure the quality of care.

Structure
Available capital facilities that meet defined standards (hospital accreditation)
Number of personnel with appropriate training
Appropriate training programmes

Accessibility
Affordability
Distance and transport facilities
Waiting lists for care

Process
Deviations from normative standards. This requires the preparation of guidelines for good practice based upon:
    Consensus conferences
    Meta-analysis of published work
    Clinical decision making
    Establishment of efficacy and effectiveness
    Definitions of appropriate care
Fragmentation vs. continuity of care
Variations in care
Imparting information and inter-personal skills
Economic assessments of effectiveness

Severity of illness
Health status before intervention

Outcome
Mortality, adjusted for case-mix severity of illness
Morbidity
    Disease-specific indices of morbidity
    Measured general health status
    Perceived health status
Satisfaction with care

Measures of structural aspects of quality

In some ways the structural aspects of the quality of care are the easiest to measure. It is easy for government departments to count the number of hospitals and to build new hospitals in areas of apparent deficiency. Such measurements of inter-regional deficiencies in structural resources in the United Kingdom led to the Resource Allocation Working Party (RAWP) in 1976, and subsequently to a more equitable distribution of structural resources. It should be easy, too, to count the number of specialists and their distribution, although in the UK this has largely been left to the specialist societies rather than the Department of Health. It is, however, less easy to define the number of specialists required. For example, neurologists in the UK have recently decided that good neurological care can be delivered by five neurologists per million population,[27] whereas representatives of the specialty in the United States of America recommend about seven times that number.[28] The criteria for deciding the compass of work of a specialist, and for how many are required, are barely explored.[29, 30]

Another way of auditing structure is by measuring how well hospitals or other structures of care match previously determined standards. This is a policy that consumes many resources in the United States, through the accreditation/certification procedures of the Joint Commission on the Accreditation of Health Care Organisations and the Health Care Financing Administration. Setting institutional standards against which care might be audited is an active endeavour of the King's Fund in the UK. The National Association of Health Authorities has also called for a National Health Service Inspectorate to ensure that all hospitals meet required standards.[31] However, Black[32] has warned that without better information than is currently available about how differently patients fare in different institutions, the role of an inspectorate or accrediting agency is likely to be limited to spotting disasters such as deficiencies in the care of the elderly mentally infirm that led in 1969 to the establishment of the Health Advisory Service.

One current way of auditing structure in the UK is through the approval of posts for general professional or higher medical training. It is mandatory, in the case of posts for training physicians, that an outside visit by a team, organised from the training office of the Royal College of Physicians, takes place not less frequently than once in ten years, while reviews can be carried out by Regional Advisers, as representatives of the College, every five years. Deficiencies in hospital facilities that influence training decide whether a post is approved as suitable for training purposes. It is difficult to document evidence of improvement of posts, as inspection only began in 1973 and initially was on an ad hoc basis. However, many Health Authorities have provided better facilities for post-graduate education and better duty rotas following suggestions that approval of their posts for training might be withdrawn. More than 1100 posts were considered by visiting teams, or by supporting documents in the year ending March 1989. Of these, 3% were not approved, and for a larger number (23%) approval was given only for a limited term. Full approval for five years was given for 75% of posts.

Measures of accessibility

Financial limitations

A general perception of inequity of access led to the establishment of the National Health Service in Britain in 1946 and of Medicare in the United States of America (USA) in 1965. Culyer[33] briefly reviews the evidence that the demand for care is, in economic terms, price elastic. In 1968, Saskatchewan introduced fees for consultations with doctors — $1.50 per surgery visit and $2.00 per house call. The average rate of use fell by 7%, and for the poor by 18%, indicating that, even with these modest charges, a significant number of people, particularly those in the low-income, high-risk group, did not seek medical care. A similar reduction in office visit rates in a health maintenance organisation occurred in 1985 when a five dollar 'co-payment' charge was required. Cherkin and colleagues[34] found that primary care visits were reduced by 10.9% and specialty visits by 3.3%. Co-payments had a greater impact on women than men aged less than 40, and on previous frequent users of primary care. Once in hospital, however, poorer people usually stay longer, and probably require more resources.[35]

In the USA, the advent of Medicare has had one surprising effect. Counter to first intuitions, one study showed that insured adults of working age in the USA had less access to care than the elderly.[36] This was not related to the different levels of need, as insured adults of working age were 3.5 times as likely as the elderly not to have received needed supportive services. The same study showed that uninsured poor, black or Hispanic people were at risk for even greater problems with access to care, and the same groups have been found to be at risk with regard to adverse outcomes of neonatal care.[37]

Geographical accessibility

Physical accessibility to care is also important, so that distance from care and adequate transport facilities are dimensions of quality. There is often a trade-off in quality between accessibility, technical competence, and effectiveness. For example, is it better to travel many miles to a well equipped radiotherapy unit, or fewer miles for less effective treatment closer to home in a less well equipped unit?[38]

Waiting

One traditional method of measuring accessibility is the number of patients waiting for treatment. Poor quality of care is reflected in the need to wait in the UK for years for, for example, some orthopaedic operations. Government in the UK is very sensitive to the length of waiting lists, but many hospitals pay insufficient regard to their accurate maintenance. If the changes proposed in the National Health Service and Community Care Bill are enacted, no hospital will be able to neglect continuous audit of its waiting list, as family doctors will take length of wait much more clearly into account when deciding where to refer patients.

Accessibility within hospitals

Accessibility *within* hospitals may also be a measure of quality. For example, are there effective systems for allowing advice to be readily obtained from senior staff, or from consultants in other specialties? For routine inpatient referrals between firms an auditable standard could be set — for example, that 70% of requests for consultation were fulfilled within 18 hours, and 95% within 48 hours. A further example of accessibility within hospitals is the positioning of defibrillators. In this case the auditable standard might be that no patient in a designated acute bed should be further than 60 seconds from a defibrillator.

Covert inaccessibility

A larger problem is covert inaccessibility to proper care because of ignorance of what is available or what is appropriate, or apathy, or possibly conscious or unconscious rationing by family doctors. For example, through the National Health Service prescribing computer, Hampton and colleagues[39] identified patients with angina in family practice by their use of nitrates, drugs used virtually only for this condition. They then reviewed the patients and showed that there was probably inappropriate under-investigation of many patients. For example, only 60% of patients had had an electrocardiogram recorded at some time, only 7% an exercise test and only 4% a coronary angiogram.

Some simple measures of access have not yet been widely employed in the UK, perhaps because they are not 'British'. For example, it is simple to telephone from outside the hospital and ascertain not only the waiting time, for example, for an orthopaedic outpatient consultation, but also the general level of timeliness of response and courtesy of the clerical staff making an appointment. In the USA such probe calls are commonplace as one method of checking the quality of the response of staff in health maintenance organisations.[40]

Measures of the quality of process of care

Donabedian[10] suggests that quality of care may be defined as the degree of conformance to, or deviation from, normative behaviour — a blunt definition within which that of Brook and Kosecoff,[8] quoted above can be subsumed.

Definition of normative standards of care

Many physicians would hold that their care is guided by the results of scientific publications in medical journals, particularly by the results of randomised clinical trials. However, it is often difficult to generalise from these — hence the interest in meta-analysis of clinical trials,[41] and in the translation of what is known about scientific medicine into clinical guidelines,[42, 42a, 42b] or the publication of the results of consensus conferences (eg 43). It has been shown that when formulating their consensus statement, those attending consensus conferences do take into account the scientific worth of contributions to the literature.[44]

Although intuitively it might be thought that the publication of consensus statements or clinical guidelines would influence clinical practice, there is as yet rather weak evidence that this is so. For example, about 90% of all obstetricians in Ontario agreed with widely circulated guidelines about the indications for Caesarian section, which if adopted would result in a substantial reduction in the rate of Caesarian section. However, two years after dissemination of the guidelines, the section rate had changed so little that, if the same

rate of change were maintained, it would take more than 30 years for
the section rate in Ontario to fall to the rate for England and Wales,
a rate generally considered to be more appropriate.[45] These relatively disappointing results should not, however, prevent us from
continuing our efforts to improve practice. The problem is how best
to change physicians' behaviour — a problem considered on p. 75.
However, as examples of the benefit to be gained, it has been shown
that patients with multiple myeloma survive significantly longer if a
treatment protocol is adhered to in preference to treatment determined by the free choice of a clinician,[16] and peri-operative hypoxic
episodes have been reduced in the United States[46] since the publication of standards for anaesthetic monitoring. In the State of
Massachusetts, malpractice insurance premiums are discounted
significantly to those anaesthetists who use a pulse oximeter on every
patient.

Some physicians object on principle to guidelines and consensus
statements, believing that such initiatives stifle research and innovative treatment. This of course is not so. No criticism could be
directed against a physician for trying innovative treatment based
upon sound research and preliminary study. Other physicians fear
that litigation may follow any departure from the guidelines. The
same argument applies. Indeed, the provision of guidelines,
especially to less experienced doctors, may lessen the frequency of
errors or omissions leading to litigation. Finally, it must of course be
remembered that although suggested procedures to be followed
may be specified by the presenting condition, what is appropriate for
a patient depends upon the individuality of that particular patient.

Regional variations in care and appropriate care

The recognition that there are startling variations in medical and
surgical practice between doctors and between geographical regions
has been a major stimulus to work on the quality of care (eg 47–50).
Table 2 illustrates the extent of regional variations in the rates of
undertaking certain surgical procedures in New England.[49] Even
allowing for the different case-mix in the two cities, a Bostonian
Medicare enrollee had in 1982 more than twice the chances of
having a carotid endarterectomy than a New Haven resident, and
only half the chances of coronary artery bypass surgery. The length
of stay for the first procedure was 30% more in Boston than in New
Haven. Although some variation in practice is of course appropriate,
as patients' needs differ, it is not possible to account for anything
other than a small amount of the variation by prevalence, severity of

Table 2. Selected types of major surgery: ratio between Boston and New Haven for Medicare patients.

	Discharges per 1,000	Length of stay
Carotid endarterectomy	2.33	1.30
Total hip replacement	1.48	1.10
Coronary bypass surgery	0.49	1.28
Hysterectomy	0.65	1.12

Data from Wennberg *et al.*[49]

illness or socio-economic factors. The variations apparently reflect differences in 'styles' of practice, independent of appropriateness of surgical interventions.

An example in variation of medical as opposed to surgical practice can be found in the UK study on transient ischaemic attacks. For the 27 neurologists entering 10 or more patients into the trial, the proportion of patients submitted to angiography varied from 3–100%![51] In the same study, the proportion of patients undergoing carotid surgery varied between 0 and 25%. The authors report:

> Either this variation (in policies in regard to investigation and surgery) makes no difference to the clinical outcome, in which case the surgical policy should be abandoned on the grounds of expense (if no other), or in some centres patients are receiving more effective (or more dangerous) treatment than in others.[51]

Perrin and Homer[50] have shown very considerable variation also in the rates of hospitalisation of children in different communities, but variations in care are not confined to hospital practice. For example, the proportion of patients referred by family doctors to hospital for specialist advice may vary twenty-fold.[52] The 'right' rate of referral cannot be known, but it is reasonable to believe that those who refer fewest patients are probably not giving their patients sufficient opportunity of specialist advice, and those who refer most are probably inefficient, in the sense of consuming excessive resources.

Measures of appropriateness of care

The best known methodology of defining appropriateness (see
above) is that developed by Brook and co-workers at the RAND
Corporation (eg 8, 18, 20). In brief, a list of possible 'indications' for
a procedure is defined, using as guides a review of the literature. The
indications categorise patients in terms of their symptoms, history
and the result of previous diagnostic tests. These indications are then
presented to panellists who rate whether it would be appropriate or
inappropriate to perform that procedure on a patient with those
indications. Ratings are made on a 9-point scale; a rating of 1 is given
if the panellist believes that the procedure is very inappropriate for
that indication, a rating of 9 for the most appropriate indication.
Discussions amongst panellists after their initial rating, followed by
re-rating, reduces the dispersion of the ratings. This is undoubtedly
a valuable technique for sharpening physicians' views on appropriateness. However, just as there may be cultural differences in normative structural standards, such as the numbers of specialists required,
so there may be in standards of appropriate procedures. For
example, for a patient with angina occurring on mild exertion (class
III), coronary artery bypass surgery was thought by a USA panel to
be appropriate, with a median rating of 7 on a 9-point scale of appropriateness, the patient being on sub-maximal medical therapy, and
with a positive exercise test. However, a panel of UK physicians and
cardiologists rated the procedure as clearly inappropriate (median
rating of 2/9).[53] Similar cultural differences have been shown in the
choice of appropriate management of neurological disease, using
rather fuller 'potted case histories' or clinical vignettes.[54]

Normative standards apply not only to technical professional practices, as listed above, but also to the setting in which the care is delivered (eg inpatient versus outpatient care) and also to factors such as
length of stay. Deviations from normative standards in relation to setting of operation and to length of stay are particularly relevant in
relation to day-care surgery, and the duration of inpatient stay after
operations of greater magnitude. Again, however, regional variations persist, even within the same system of health care (Table 2).

Inappropriate admission, investigations and procedures all consume resources that could be applied to appropriate care. Even if
initial hospitalisation is appropriate, patients may stay unnecessarily
long in hospital, through inertia or ineffective practice, waiting for
investigations or procedures, or waiting for arrangements to be
made for their discharge. Using a set of standardised criteria, a number of studies have shown that between 12% and 28% of hospital

days are inappropriate.[55-57] A striking example of variation in practice comes from Wennberg's further analysis of hospitalisation rates in Boston and New Haven.[58] Without in this case making judgements about appropriateness, Wennberg and colleagues found that 40% of all deaths occurred in hospital in Boston, and 32% in New Haven. Assuming similar overall illness rates (and there were low variations in admission rates for some marker conditions such as coronary artery disease), there was no discernible difference in survival between the two cities, associated with an 80% difference in Medicare reimbursements. Wennberg remarks that a study of different approaches to the treatment of medical conditions with high variation in admission rates (eg diabetes, chronic obstructive airways disease) should have priority on our research agenda.

Most of the studies quoted in this review refer to inpatient care. However, inappropriate investigation may also occur in outpatient practice. I give two examples from my own specialty of neurology. After a first seizure (usually a tonic-clonic convulsion in adults) it has been traditional to perform an electroencephalogram (EEG) and in the last fifteen years, a cranial CT scan. However, a prospective study of more than 400 patients aged 16 or over showed that changes in the EEG did not predict seizure recurrence, and the data suggested that a cranial CT scan is only necessary in occasional clearly defined circumstances.[59] The second example concerns multiple sclerosis. A number of investigations are available to support what is essentially a clinical diagnosis. These include lumbar puncture, evoked visual, brainstem or somatosensory responses, and magnetic resonance imaging. A careful analysis will show which, if any, are appropriate in any particular case.[60] I believe that such research studies and analyses are a better foundation for the judgement of appropriateness than the views of panels which, as described above, may differ strikingly according to the composition of the panel.[53]

Does inappropriate use explain regional variations?

Implicit in many of the publications on regional variations in the use of medical and surgical procedures is the assumption that high rates of use are the result of the more frequent application of inappropriate procedures. Unfortunately, this attractive explanation appears to be only partly true. Brook's group at the RAND Corporation has shown that for coronary angiography in counties with high use rates, patients were more likely to be investigated inappropriately; even so, across counties, inappropriate use accounted for only 28% of the variance in use rates. However, there was no correlation between rates of use and appropriateness across counties for upper gastro-intestinal endoscopy or carotid endarterectomy.[60a] Brook and colleagues suggest that local variations in incidence of disease between counties is quite insufficient to account for the variation in rates of use, nor did the RAND group find any evidence that counties had a general propensity to use all procedures at high or low rates — a county might have a high incidence rate for endoscopy, but a low rate for carotid endarterectomy. These findings suggest that the RAND's ratings of appropriateness may be too lax. As the authors write: 'It is possible that a process that rated an indication appropriate only when there was evidence of effectiveness from a controlled clinical trial might have resulted in a stronger relationship between rate of use and appropriateness'. It would be interesting to repeat this study using the more restrained criteria of appropriateness of British practice, examples of which have already been cited.[53, 54]

Clinical decision making

An alternative to consensus judgements of appropriateness, and another dimension by which deviations from normative practice can be measured, is founded upon clinical decision making. For this is required a basic knowledge of probability theory. In order to assess the odds of being affected, given a positive result of an investigation or the presence of a certain illness feature, it is necessary to know the prevalence of the disease in the community, and the specificity, sensitivity and rate of false positives of the clinical feature elicited, or the investigation under consideration.[61]

Clinical decision making extends beyond diagnosis to strategies of management. It should take into account the probabilities of different outcomes of different clinical actions, the probabilities of risks and benefits associated with these actions, and an analysis of how the patient's interests, and preferences should best be served.[62–64] In this context, the utility of the outcome is an assessment of the preferences of those involved in making the decision about an action — including the patient, his family, physician and society. As Eddy[65] writes, clinicians must adjust so that

> instead of a simple qualitative judgement that a procedure may have a benefit, a quantitative estimate must be made about the magnitude of the benefit,' and secondly that instead of focusing only on the patient when making a decision, the scope of the decision must be broadened

to include comparison across procedures and diseases, and 'attention to the efficiency, yield and priority of different activities.

Howard[66] has considered the problem of explaining to patients probabilities of different outcomes of treatment. He points out that a scale of probability of 0 to 1 is inconvenient, as many of the clinical probabilities to be considered are small. No-one, he writes, would discuss a rug measuring 0.00170 miles × 0.00227 miles. His solution is to use microprobability units of 1 in a million. When the risk consequence is death, he proposes an intriguingly named unit — the 'micromort'. For example, the annual probability of death due to a motor accident in the USA is 270 micromorts, or approximately 5 micromorts a week. For comparison, the assessed risk of dying as a result of a cerebral angiogram performed for the investigation of a suspected angioma is 1 in 600 or 1,600 micromorts — more than 300 times the risks of living with motor vehicles for one week, a much more readily understandable risk.

Balla and colleagues[64] point out that many doctors feel uneasy with information about probabilities. They have psychological perceptions of occurrence and of risk which are influenced by their own recent experience and specialty, and which are not based upon the scientific literature. For example, surgeons will first think of gall-stones as an explanation for jaundice, physicians hepatitis or drug-induced liver damage. Furthermore, doctors tend to overestimate the probabilities of salient and vivid events, perhaps here at one with patients who have been shown to be very risk-averse towards taking chances involving their health[67] (see p. 45). Nonetheless, it is probable that in the next decade the familiar published algorithms for the management of some common conditions[68] will be replaced by decision trees, in which the nodal points will be marked by estimates of the *expected value* (also called the *expected utility*) of each management option. The expected value is calculated by multiplying probability and utility.

At times we may choose an action with a low probability outcome provided that the outcome has a high utility, and the other branch, even if it had a higher probability outcome, has a low utility. We are looking for high *expected values* of management strategies. An example of a decision tree is shown in Fig. 2. Such decision trees could be used for audit, and for education. Medical care which consistently followed pathways with low expected value would clearly be of poor quality. In Fig. 2, the utility of stroke and death is considered to be of higher utility in the aspirin treated group, as these two outcomes may occur immediately after surgery, but are likely to be

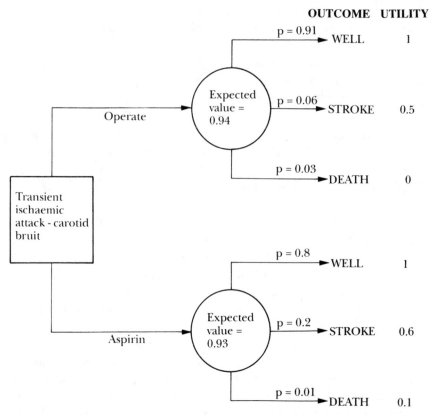

OUTCOME   UTILITY

Fig. 2. *Illustration of decision tree used in clinical decision analysis.* The utility of stroke and death is considered to be higher in the group treated by aspirin than the group subjected to carotid endarterectomy, since if stroke or death are associated with surgery, they are likely to occur soon after the intervention. (Figure kindly provided by Professor J.I. Balla.)

delayed for those treated medically and so can be discounted (p. 50). It is possible to test the stability of our conclusions about the expected value of alternative strategies by putting other plausible estimates of utility and probability into the tree.

The Journal of the American Medical Association has just started a regular column on clinical decision making.[68a] In the first article, Eddy[68b] reviews the extraordinary variations in the *beliefs* of specialists about the probability of different outcomes, a variation which must go some way to explain variations in clinical practice (see p. 16). One way to reduce such variation is to encourage the widespread use of probabilities of outcome derived from the literature, and widespread discussion as to the appropriate evaluation of utilities.

Fragmentation versus continuity of care

In the management of complex illnesses, the skills of a number of different specialists and their assistants may be required, and patients understand and value this. However, in established, chronic illnesses, patient satisfaction surveys show that they also value continuity of supportive management. This is an aspect that can readily be audited. For example, some years ago in one community study of epilepsy,[68c] a patient had attended a world famous hospital 22 times and seen 16 different doctors, but never the consultant responsible for his care.

Imparting information and interpersonal skills

Communication is a two-way business. All too often in clinical practice a physician believes that he has made every effort to communicate to a patient and his relatives a diagnosis and plan of management, only to hear later that the patient has complained that 'the doctor didn't tell me anything.' Many studies rank failure of communication as a leading cause of patient dissatisfaction (see p. 55 *et seq.*). An extensive body of literature exists in the field (for references see 69, 70).

Bourhis and colleagues[70] have recently underlined how doctors are 'bi-lingual', speaking both 'medical' and 'everyday' language. Their study showed that doctors attempted to use everyday language (but were not rated by nurses as being very successful at it), and also that patients attempted to use medical language, but were not encouraged to do so by the doctors. A confounding problem seemed to be that 'because doctors use medical language every day, it may become in some way an everyday language'— that is to say, doctors may find it difficult to differentiate between everyday and medical language when talking to patients. An interesting approach to this problem has been adopted by Tattersall, a diabetologist in the UK.[71] After each outpatient visit, he writes to the referring general practitioner, as all of us do, but he also sends a copy to the patient. This means that the letter has to be written in jargon-free terms. In effect, although Tattersall does not explicitly state this, he is trying to revert to the use of everyday language even when communicating with doctors.

Quill[72] has recently reviewed some of the barriers that arise in doctor–patient communication, and ways of recognising and surmounting them. Another recent study stresses the differences between the lexical and grammatical content of *what* a doctor says and the vocal component of *how* it is said. Harrigan and colleagues[73] review how greater weight is given to vocal cues when interpreting contradictory verbal and vocal messages.

Although an active research field, medical students receive little instruction in communication. Young doctors appear to develop a style which reflects the strengths and weaknesses of their own personality, often modelled upon a charismatic 'powerful' teacher, thus perpetuating physician dominance in physician–patient interaction.

Measures of deviation from normative standards

Deviation from normative standards of care traditionally has been detected by physicians working together in one hospital, particularly in the framework of a consultant teaching his registrar, or by friendly analysis of case-management in the context of 'Grand Rounds'. However, the view has developed, particularly in the USA, that the degree of conformance to normative standards of care can at present only be judged by reference to the written medical record. The weakness of such a system of audit of course is that excellent humane medical care can be given by a doctor who writes appalling records; conversely, complaints may be made by patients that 'he never even looked at me, he was too busy writing.' However, review of good practice by reference to the written record is now the established system of medical audit in the USA, and, as such, is briefly reviewed here.

Peer review organisations (PROs)

The detection of deviation from normative standards of care is the basis for the vast Peer Review Organisation (PRO) and commercial medical audit systems that have become necessary in the USA. Section 1156 of the Social Security Act places a statutory obligation on providers and practitioners who provide health care services for which payment will in whole or in part be made by Medicare to assure that services or items ordered:

— will be provided economically and only when, and to the extent, medically necessary

— will be of a quality which meets professionally recognised standards of health care

— will be supported by evidence of medical necessity and quality in such form and fashion and at such time as may reasonably be required by a reviewing peer review organisation in the exercise of its duties and responsibilities.

A PRO is contracted to the Health Care Financing Administration (HCFA) to undertake these responsibilities. The method that a PRO employs is for a registered nurse chart (medical record) reviewer to evaluate the written record, or photocopies of it, against normative standard protocols. For example, using an 'Admission Evaluation Protocol', the reviewer will determine whether care might as well have been provided in a nursing home or as an outpatient. Reviewers also check for unnecessary prolongation of inpatient care, and check the record for the clinical information that led to assignation to a Diagnosis Related Group (DRG). PRO reviewers check other aspects of the quality of process of care, against so called 'generic quality screens' some of which are listed in Table 3.

The peer review organisation in the State of Massachusetts, MassPRO, finds that about 20% of selected records will fail the quality screen and be referred to a medical reviewer, who, using his clinical judgement, may decide that the failure was a 'technical' screen failure, and does not reflect a real failure of quality. In the six months period from March to September 1988, 2.1% of all charts reviewed did reveal a failure of quality confirmed by a physician.[74]

Common failures of quality revealed by the PRO screens include misuse of antibiotics, particularly lack of care in prescribing amino-glycosides, a failure to use antibiotics in accord with laboratory-determined sensitivities, and sloppy writing of prescriptions in general. Failure to seek specialist advice when appropriate, and unnecessary fragmentation of care are also common faults.

Identification of a doctor's failures of quality may result in a 'corrective action plan', directed at educating the doctor. For example, it may be mandatory for some months for a surgeon to seek a further opinion before operating on a class of patients. Although the PROs strive to convince physicians that they serve an educational function, many physicians regard their actions as intrusive and potentially punitive, as their final sanction is to withhold Medicare payment. Other criticisms include the fact that many failures of quality are random, and as such, do not appear in the 'screens', and may remain undetected by the chart reviewers. Retrospective chart review is untimely in so far as it cannot influence the care of the individual patient. The need to satisfy PRO requirements divert staff from assessing and assuring other aspects of quality. Moreover, many physicians feel that the PRO system is a cost-inefficient way of detecting failures of quality. MassPRO, for example, has a budget of approximately 7 million dollars. It employs a full-time medical director, four associate directors, and 70 medical record (chart) reviewers, who are registered nurses. In the year ending March 1989,

Table 3. Generic quality screen for inpatients.

---

*1. **Adequacy of discharge planning**
No documentation of discharge planning or appropriate followup care with consideration of physical, emotional, and mental status needs at time of discharge

2. **Medical stability of the patient at discharge**
   a. BP within 24 hours of discharge (systolic less than 85 or greater than 180; diastolic less than 50 or greater than 110)
   b. Temperature within 24 hours of discharge greater than 101 degrees Fahrenheit (38.3 Centigrade) oral, greater than 102 degrees Fahrenheit (38.9 Centigrade) rectal
   c. Pulse less than 50 (or 45 if the patient is on a beta blocker), or greater than 120 within 24 hours of discharge
   d. Abnormal diagnostic findings which are not addressed and resolved or where the record does not explain why they are not resolved
   e. Intravenous fluids or drugs after 12 midnight on day of discharge
   f. Purulent or bloody drainage of wound or open area within 24 hours prior to discharge

3. **Deaths**
   a. During or following any surgery performed during the current admission
   b. Following return to intensive care unit, coronary care or other special care unit within 24 hours of being transferred out.
   c. Other unexpected death

*4. **Nosocomial infection**
Hospital acquired infection

5. **Unscheduled return to surgery**
Within same admission for same condition as previous surgery or to correct operative problem

6. **Trauma suffered in hospital**
   a. Unplanned surgery which includes, but is not limited to, removal or repair of a normal organ or body part (ie surgery not addressed specifically in the operative consent)
   *b. Fall
   c. Serious complications of anaesthesia
   d. Any transfusion error or serious transfusion reaction
   * e. Hospital acquired decubitus ulcer and/or deterioration of an existing decubitus
   f. Medication error or adverse drug reaction (1) with serious potential for harm or (2) resulting in measures to correct
   g. Care or lack of care resulting in serious or potentially serious complications

Optional screen
Medication or treatment changes (including discontinuation) within 24 hours of discharge without adequate observation

---

* PRO reviewer is to record the failure of the screen, but need not refer potential severity Level I quality problems to physician reviewer until a pattern emerges.

Data from US Department of Health and Human Services, Health Care Financing Administration, Health Standards and Quality Bureau. (Reproduced with kind permission.)

MassPRO reviewed 238,917 hospital discharges (115,618 cases).[74] The cost per record reviewed varied between 45 and 80 dollars.

Record review in the United Kingdom

A much simpler form of record review has been proposed in the UK.[5] It is suggested that notes are randomly selected and reviewed at short intervals by physician(s) other than the one under whose care the patient has been admitted. Table 4 lists the headings under which the process of care as recorded in the hospital notes is audited.

Such audit has been shown to improve immensely the quality of the written record.[75] It has now been agreed by the Royal College of Physicians that when a team visits a district to inspect the suitability of posts, a random selection of notes will be reviewed in this way, and upon their quality will depend the recognition of the post as suitable for training.

Utilisation review

Another way in which adherence to normative standards is controlled in the USA is by preadmission review.[76] Under the PRO system, before a surgeon can proceed with, for example, a hip replacement in Massachusetts, he must satisfy a reviewer, by a telephone call, that the patient fulfils certain conditions related to degree of disability and clinical findings.

Similar utilisation reviews are now operated by many health care insurers. For example, an insured person is required, through his physicians, to obtain by telephone certification of the appropriateness of his planned admission, and, when in hospital, certification of the appropriateness of his continuing stay and plan of treatment. Utilisation review was originally required by the insurers of large corporate and union customers but has now extended to individual subscribers in some companies.[77] If pre-admission certification is not obtained, the portion of the patient's expenses covered by insurance may be reduced by 10% or more, although physicians and other health care providers are not subject to such penalties. Table 5 is an extract from a pamphlet produced by Empire Blue Cross and Blue Shield (New York) Managed Care Program.

By analysing insurance claims data on more than 200 groups of employees, Feldstein and colleagues were able to show that utilisation review reduced admissions by an average of 12.3%, inpatient days by 8.0%, and hospital expenditures by 11.9%. The ratio of savings to the costs of the review programme was very favourable —

Table 4. Suggested form for use of visiting Fellows when auditing case notes.[5]

Consultant:...   Date: ....
Auditor:..

> **Patient's name and details are NOT to be included
> in order to maintain strict confidentiality**

FINAL DIAGNOSIS: ....
....
....

A. DETAILS OF ADMISSION

 i Source of admission:

   a Emergency take.................................   Bed Bureau ....

   b Waiting list of O.P.............................   G.P. ....

   c Other ....

 ii Is there evidence to suggest a delay in admission? Yes/No

   If so, at what stage?...
....

 iii Do the notes indicate what drugs patient was taking on admission? Yes/No
....

B. DOCUMENTATION OF ILLNESS

 i Were initial medical notes adequate? Yes/No
....

 ii Were the clinical problems clearly set out? Yes/No
....

 iii Was the subsequent course of the illness well documented? Yes/No
....

 iv Were notes signed and dated? Yes/No
....

continued

C. PATIENT EDUCATION AND WELFARE

i Is it clear from the notes what discussions took place and what information was given to:

a Patients? Yes/No

....

b Relatives? Yes/No

....

ii Is it clear whether the GP was consulted about admission, management or discharge? Yes/No

....

D. DISCHARGE

i **House physician's letter**

How many days after discharge was it sent?

Does it contain adequate information about:

a Diagnosis? Yes/No

....

b Discharge medication? Yes/No

....

c Patient information? Yes/No

d Follow-up arrangements? Yes/No

....

e Request for domiciliary services, if appropriate? Yes/No

....

ii **Case notes summary**

How many days after discharge was it sent?

Was documentation of admission adequate? Yes/No

....

Was drug therapy clearly stated? Yes/No

....

Was it clear what information was given to patient and relatives? Yes/No

....

Are follow-up plans clearly stated and appropriate? Yes/No

....

E. GENERAL COMMENTS

....
....
....
....

Table 5. Extract from conditions imposed by Empire Blue Cross and Blue Shield Managed care.

Remember, the final decision whether or not to have surgery is yours. Failure to obtain a second opinion prior to undergoing any of the procedures listed in the second opinion procedure list will result in a reduction of your benefits by 10%. If, in our judgement, the procedure was not medically necessary, benefits may be denied in full.

Second Opinion on Surgery List

- back surgery (limited to disc surgery, including disc injection therapy, laminectomy and/or infusion)
- gall bladder surgery (limited to removal of gall bladder for stones)
- heart surgery (limited to surgery for coronary artery disease)
- hip surgery (limited to total replacement)
- hysterectomy (partial or total removal of uterus)
- prostatectomy (partial or total removal of prostate)
- carotid artery surgery (carotid endarterectomy)

Reproduced by kind permission.[77]

about 8:1.[76] Another publication reported very similar findings.[78] Rosenberg and colleagues have studied patients' reactions to utilisation review prior to surgery.[79] Most patients felt that a further opinion before surgery provided reassurance and helped decide whether to have the operation. Many also felt that the additional consultation provided a chance to ask important questions. Few patients reported that an additional consultation caused anxiety or provoked confusion, and the advice of the second consultant was discordant with that of the first in only 21 of 537 instances (3.9%). Interestingly, however, patients sometimes reported discordant advice, even when the second consultant's written report was concordant with the first. Discordance was more likely if the patients themselves rated the consultants who provided the second opinions as not thorough and understandable when explaining their opinions and answering questions.

Pre-admission and utilisation review have until recently depended upon concordant opinions of colleagues, or upon the fulfilment of simple criteria laid down by medical advisers to a PRO or insurance company (eg Table 5). However, workers at the RAND Corporation have, by more organised evaluations of what is appropriate (eg ref 18), established criteria that should be fulfilled before a procedure is undertaken. Kosecoff has demonstrated a micro-computer based system that allows a nurse or physician reviewer to question over the telephone the appropriateness of a physician's request for a procedure, based upon ratings of appropriateness of panels informed by a literature review. About ten million Americans are now covered by insurance plans that require such pre-procedural review of appropriateness.[80]

4 | Outcomes of care

Mortality rates

Population mortality

Perinatal and neonatal mortality rates have for years been used as an index of the health and provision of medical care to large populations. The enormous decline in these indices since data were first collected may fairly be taken as evidence of improved quality of housing, of general sanitary standards and of medical care. However, the rate of decline is now flattening out, approaching perhaps a figure at which genetic and other (at present) unavoidable factors are predominant. In developed countries, the index has become therefore relatively insensitive to the quality of care, although remaining large differences between blacks and whites in the USA continue to point to unacceptable differences in quality of care.

Avoidable mortality can be used as a measure of the quality of care delivered to populations. Rutstein and colleagues[81] have published a table of index causes of death which are at least potentially avoidable. These include deaths associated with smoking, inadequate immunisation rates, and alcohol related and other road traffic accidents. Geographical variations in avoidable mortality have been published by Charlton and colleagues,[82, 83] and the data is also available in atlas form. Mackenbach and colleagues[84] have reviewed the differences in mortality between socio-economic groups in England and Wales, and concluded that a widening in the differences over the last few decades (1931–81) was partly due to differences in decline of mortality from conditions amenable to medical intervention, which in turn were due, at least in part, to differences between socio-economic groups in accessibility, utilisation or quality of medical care.

Hospital mortality

'Differences in patient death rates seem on their face a valid way to distinguish good quality health care providers from poor quality providers; death is an outcome that is almost always bad, and medical practice is devoted, at least in part, to postponing death.'[85] This quotation is a succinct introduction to the use of mortality rates as a valid indicator of the quality of hospital medical care. However, the literature on differences in hospital mortality is generally unsatisfactory.

Brook and colleagues[86] reviewed the available literature, calling particular attention to the most frequently mentioned difficulty — the relative inability to measure differences between patients that might affect death rates. Principal among these differences is of course age, but obviously the severity of the illness for which admission is required is also a major determinant of outcome, as are co-existent illnesses ('co-morbidities').

Iezzoni writes that 'an entire industry has arisen to define and measure the severity of illness of hospitalised patients.'[87] She reviews the historical background leading up to the need to rate severity, and some of the more successful attempts to do so. She also points out that definitions of severity depend upon the perspective from which it is viewed. An acute surgical crisis may severely threaten the life of the patient, but, by the time a month has passed, the patient may again be perfectly well. Conversely, the management of a hemiplegia may not consume many resources because the patient may stay at home — but this is a severe illness from the patient's perspective as his whole quality of life has changed. The development of most measures of severity has, however, been on acute illnesses, as, in the US health system where these have been developed, the accent is on the possibility of relating severity of illness to hospital charges. Although Diagnosis Related Groups (DRGs), the basis of the Prospective Payment System, do reflect severity across DRGs, they cannot reflect severity within DRGs.

There are five well-known systems of measuring severity of illness — the Acute Physiology and Chronic Health Evaluation systems (APACHE II),[88] the Computerised Severity Index (Health Systems International), Disease Staging by clinical criteria and Q scale (SysteMetrics), MedisGroups, and Patient Management Categories (Pittsburgh Research Institute). The concepts and methodologies of these are reviewed by Iezzoni.[87]

Predicted outcome (mortality) adjusted for severity of illness can be used as an audit measure. Three examples follow.

Knaus and colleagues[89] used the APACHE score — a score of illness based upon a limited number of physiological and clinical variables[88] — to compare the number of observed deaths compared with the number of predicted deaths in 13 hospitals. One hospital, for example, did very well with 69 predicted deaths, but only 41 observed. Another hospital had significantly worse results with 58%

more deaths than the number predicted. Knaus and colleagues[89] found that the variations reflected the different degrees of co-ordination of intensive care rather than other variables, such as whether the hospital was a teaching centre or not. It has been pro-posed[90] that similar methods be used for audit of neonatal intensive care units. However, Pollack and colleagues[91] found that differences in mortality amongst children in intensive care could be explained by differences in illness severity and age alone.

The Health Care Financing Administration (HCFA) collects data about deaths occurring within 30 days of admission of Medicare patients.[92] Adjustments are made for age, sex, co-morbidities tailored to diagnostic group, previous health as measured by prior hospital admissions in the year preceding death, and whether a patient was transferred from another hospital. The data is published in complex tables from which can be read outlying hospitals with a significantly higher or lower mortality. As Berwick[93] has pointed out 'the hun-dreds of pages of data are dwarfed by the thousand pages of responses from hospitals, trying to prove whatever hospitals need to prove to build their defenses.'

Many in the United States have argued that the HCFA data do not adequately allow for illness severity. Green and colleagues[93a] have recently shown that the HCFA model has a very limited capacity to predict mortality after admission to hospital. However, adding a measure of severity of illness (The Severity of Illness Index), a simple four-level ordinal scale, substantially increased the predictive power of the mathematical model and reduced instances of higher than expected hospital mortality to chance levels.

Dubois and colleagues[94, 95] reviewed 377 medical records from twelve hospitals at the extremes of the HCFA mortality statistics, before adjustment for severity of illness ('outliers'). The records chosen were for patients dying after cerebrovascular accident, myo-cardial infarction and pneumonia. After adjusting for severity of illness, the death rate in the high outliers exceeded by 3–10% that predicted from severity of illness alone. In the low outliers, the rate fell short of the severity-adjusted predictions by 10–15%. However, a review of 125 indicators of process of care failed to reveal any differ-ences between high and low outliers. Furthermore, these chosen indicators of process missed one clearly avoidable death, due to a nasogastric tube being passed into a bronchus. When professional consensus was used to judge whether any deaths had been avoidable, it was thought that 5.7% of deaths of a typical cohort could have been prevented in the high outliers, as opposed to 3.2% in the low outliers.

In a further analysis of the work cited earlier,[95] Dubois and Brook pointed out that if each preventable death had its own separate cause, then it would be very difficult for a hospital to reduce its rate of preventable deaths. However, a small number of factors were associated with most preventable deaths — in the case of myocardial infarction, less than vigorous management of unstable angina, inadequate management of fluids, inadequate haemodynamic monitoring and inadequate control of arrhythmias. For preventable stroke deaths, a review panel thought that errors in diagnosis were on the whole more relevant than errors in management.

Several themes emerged from the literature review of Dubois, Brook and colleagues:[94] that mortality tended to be lower in hospitals with committed staff who communicated well, who were board certified, and who undertook procedures frequently. Size and teaching status were also associated with lower inpatient mortality. Hartz and colleagues have also explored the structural characteristics of hospitals and their relation to mortality, using the 1986 HCFA data. They found that the adjusted mortality rate was most closely associated with the level of training of the medical staff, lower rates being associated with a higher percentage of board-certified specialists.[94a] Lower adjusted mortality rates were also associated with higher payroll expenses per hospital bed, teaching hospitals, private non-profit making hospitals, and hospitals with a higher proportion of registered nurses, a higher level of technical sophistication and larger size. Higher adjusted mortality rates were associated with osteopathic and private profit-making hospitals. We may fairly say that these variables are intuitively recognised by patients, who, at least in the UK, commonly seek opinions from large albeit inconveniently placed metropolitan teaching hospitals.

Adverse outcomes

As the preceding paragraphs show, mortality is, in general, an insensitive measure of quality of care. There is, however, one exception — and that is death occurring in circumstances where it is clearly highly unusual — for example, after a herniorrhaphy. This is an example of the general class of designated 'adverse outcomes' as markers of the quality of care. Table 6 shows some of the adverse outcomes that can be used as indicators of the quality of care.

Peri-operative or peri-procedural death

It is a requirement in the UK that such deaths are reported to the coroner. Of course the vast majority of peri-operative deaths are

Table 6. Some adverse outcomes as indicators of care of possibly low quality.

Peri-operative or peri-procedural death

Resuscitation from peri-operative or peri-procedural cardiopulmonary arrest

Deaths from potentially remediable conditions

— status epilepticus

— diabetic ketoacidosis

— extradural haematoma

Unplanned removal, injury or repair of tissue during surgery or invasive procedure

Unplanned return to operating theatre

Hospital acquired infections

Problems with drugs

— error in prescribing noted by pharmacy or another doctor

— inappropriate use of antibiotics

— inadequate care when using aminoglycosides

— prescription of drugs with known interactions

Problems with infusions

— inadequate specification or calculation of fluid/electrolytes

— unnecessary infusions

— tissue infiltration

Problems with transfusions

— unnecessary transfusion

— transfusion reaction

Abnormal result of investigation on which no appropriate action has been taken

Development of pressure sores

Falls and other injuries to patients

Complaints by patients or their relatives

Litigation

---

unavoidable, and are due to the severity or progession of the disease process for which the operation was being undertaken — for example, ruptured aortic aneurysm, or carcinoma of the head of the pancreas. However, an institutional review of all peri-operative deaths may reveal, for example, that a surgeon is operating inappropriately in patients already doomed by disseminated malignant disease, or that operations are being performed by surgeons with insufficient training or experience.[96]

Deaths from potentially remediable conditions

Patients admitted in diabetic keto-acidosis or in status epilepticus should in general not die if the urgency of the situation is recognised, and appropriate treatment given. Other examples include patients with pneumococcal meningitis, or staphylococcal or gram-negative septicaemia.

Unplanned removal or injury of normal tissue during surgery or invasive procedure

Examples here would include injury to a ureter during a hysterectomy.

Unplanned return to operating theatre

Intra-abdominal bleeding or wound dehiscence may be taken as examples of technical skills of poor quality.

A reader, especially a surgical reader, may at this point feel that the proposed use of such indicators does not recognise the skills and complexities of his work, and the problems encountered when operating upon desperately ill and often very old people. Physicians, too, are well aware of the high mortality of, for example, pneumococcal meningitis in the elderly. However, the whole purpose of medical audit is to try and identify failures in the system the resolution of which might improve the quality of care. For example, a review of peri-operative deaths in three Health Regions in the UK showed that in a number of cases junior surgeons were operating beyond their level of training, often at night, and often without seeking their advice of their senior colleagues.[96] A study of deaths from diabetic keto-acidosis or pneumococcal meningitis may well reveal similar remediable deficiencies on the medical wards.

Hospital acquired infections

About 6% of all admissions are complicated by hospital-acquired (nosocomial) infections, most commonly in surgical wards and intensive therapy units. The most common sites for infection are the urinary tract, operative wounds, and lungs. There are, however, considerable difficulties in using the incidence of hospital-acquired infection as an indicator of the quality of care. For surgical wound infections, for example, one surgeon may regard some redness and induration around the incision as nothing untoward, another classify it as a clear cut infection. There is also the point that the better the care from the point of view of investigating unexplained fevers, culturing the urine etc, the greater will be the rate of reported infections. An uncaring hospital may in contrast report a low rate.

Problems with drugs

Errors in prescriptions by junior doctors are often pointed out, with varying degrees of delicacy, by experienced nursing staff, and no record of the error is made. A hospital pharmacy, however, could readily monitor errors in dosage and the prescription of incompatible drugs.

The occurrence of allergic skin reactions can be monitored. In some cases it is found that a drug has been prescribed even though it had been recorded that the patient was sensitive to it.

Antibiotics are often used inappropriately. There are particular problems with aminoglycosides, as blood levels are taken insufficiently frequently, or the dose not altered according to the result. On other occasions antibiotics are given prophylactically before a procedure but unnecessarily, on yet others they are omitted when, as in the case of rheumatic heart disease or Caesarian section,[97] they should be given. Or they may be reasonably started on account of overt infection, before the results of culture are available, and then not changed according to the reported sensitivities.

Problems with infusions and transfusions

The frequency with which an infusion line requires replacement or 'tissues' is one measure of the technical skill with which it is inserted. An audit of ongoing infusions may reveal inadequate specification to the nursing staff of the fluid and electrolyte requirement. Some transfusions may be judged inappropriate by peer review.[98] A transfusion reaction may indicate a laboratory failure in cross-matching, or a failure in the system of labelling of blood.

Failure to address an abnormal result of investigation

The rapid turnover of patients means that the results of some investigations are returned to the ward after the patient has left hospital. Occasionally, multiple serum analyses turn up a positive result, for example hyperglycaemia, in a patient admitted for some other reason, and the abnormal result is lost sight of in the general concentration on the primary reason for admission. Failure to take appropriate action in such circumstances clearly indicates poor care.

Unplanned readmissions

There has been some interest in using the rate of unplanned re-admission of patients as a measure of the quality of care of a medical firm or hospital — on the thesis that an unplanned readmission within, say, 30 days may indicate either premature discharge or a failure to organise appropriate care in the community. However, as Henderson and colleagues point out, such a measure is fraught with methodological pit-falls.[99] The decision to readmit is influenced not only by the patient's clinical state, but by the availability of beds and the clinician's threshold for admission. There are also problems if a patient is readmitted to a hospital in another district which may not be counted unless data are collected across districts. Finally, if the rate of unplanned readmission is used as a quality measure, there is concern that trial discharges of elderly people to see if they can manage at home will be discouraged.

Unanticipated admission after day surgery

It might be thought that pressure on beds could lead to the unsafe use of day surgery. An interesting study from the United States has shown that the most common reasons for unplanned post-operative admission were pain, vomiting and bleeding. The patients' pre-operative characteristics were relatively unimportant, suggesting that there were few failures of adequate patient selection.[99a]

Pressure sores; falls and other injuries to patients

With a sufficient number of adequately trained nursing staff, and a sufficient supply of nursing aids such as low-air loss beds, pressure sores should not occur. The problem of falls is, however, more complex. For an elderly person, a degree of autonomy in, for example, getting to the lavatory unaided is a component of a life of reasonable quality. A hospital or nursing home which encourages this may provide better quality care, at some accepted risk to the patients, than another which encourages restraint with sedative drugs, cot-sides, and much nursing assistance to prevent falls. Nevitt and colleagues[100] and Morse and colleagues[101] provide guidance as to those particularly at risk for falls, and audit could be directed at whether those risk factors had been documented, and appropriate nursing procedures worked out and communicated to all staff.

Complaints

Complaints, if found to be justified on review, are clearly adverse outcomes. Even if not justified, they must imply a failure of communication. They are further considered on p. 55.

The relation between experience and outcome

Physicians and surgeons of experience may reasonably be predicted to have better outcomes than those with lesser experience. As already mentioned, the report of the Confidential Enquiry on Perioperative Deaths in the UK[96] showed clearly that many apparently avoidable peri-operative deaths followed surgery undertaken by doctors in training who had not consulted their senior colleagues, and often at night. The anaesthetists associated were, in general, also at an inappropriately early stage in their training.

Experience includes not only training, but also the passage of years, and, in the case of technical procedures or operations, the effects of practice. Studies in the USA have shown that complex surgical procedures are often undertaken by surgeons with little experience in that procedure. For example, 75% of all surgeons undertaking carotid endarterectomy on a Medicare population did less than ten endarterectomies a year, and 24% did only one. Leape and colleagues write, with some restraint, that 'Few would regard that as sufficient to maintain surgical skills.'[102] Not surprisingly, there is good evidence to support the view that the annual number of procedures ('volume') undertaken by a surgeon is related to the outcome of the procedure.

Hannan and colleagues have studied the interactions between individual surgeon volume and total hospital volume.[103] They found that for coronary artery bypass surgery, resection of an abdominal aortic aneurysm, partial gastrectomy and colectomy, the volume of operations undertaken by an individual surgeon was more important than the total hospital volume. For cholecystectomy, hospital volume was more important than the volume of operations undertaken by individual surgeons. Hannan *et al.* suggest that for this less risky procedure, the surgical team, hospital equipment and monitoring procedures are more important than the expertise of an individual surgeon. Hannan and colleagues from their data calculated threshold hospital volumes beyond which mortality rates remained more or less constant — 5 partial gastrectomies, 40 colectomies and 170 cholecystectomies. There was no detectable threshold for coronary artery bypass surgery and for abdominal aneurysms, mortality rates continuing to decline with increasing volume.

Variation in outcome between surgeons is likely to be an important audit tool in the UK. For example, in the Lothian district, it was found that mortality after operations for abdominal aortic aneurysms varied between surgeons.[104] Once the data had been collected, the surgical service was re-organised so that three surgeons specialising in vascular surgery worked together in one unit, to which other teams could refer vascular cases. There is nothing new in this. In 1914 Codman wrote

> . . . the surgical staff at the Massachusetts General Hospital did this: they re-organised in such a way that each active member of the staff undertook to give special study to some difficult class of cases, and in return the hospital assigned to each member all the cases of that group. The result has been that the mortality in these groups of cases showed a great improvement . . . .[105]

Although most of the published literature on volume and outcome relates to surgery, there is clear evidence from other fields that high volume and experience result in more favourable outcomes. Specialised spinal units, for example, have paraplegic patients with fewer pressure sores and urinary infections than ordinary hospital wards, and achieve a better final functional status for their patients. Units with greater experience of AIDS have better outcomes for patients with *Pneumocystis carinii* pneumonia than units with less experience.[106]

Outcomes of care measured by a change in health status

Apart from death and the other adverse outcomes just considered, the effectiveness and quality of care can in part be measured by changes in health status. For many acute illnesses of younger adult life the patient can fortunately expect return to a completely normal life. Examples include the resolution of acute lobar pneumonia or cystitis. Outcome measures for such diseases are more or less self-evident — the relief of symptoms, supported, if required, by investigation — in these examples the clearing of opacification on a chest X-ray, or the absence of any bacterial growth on urine culture. Such clearly defined outcomes can be comparatively easily linked to the process of care given during the acute illness, and in these examples there is no doubt of the effectiveness of anti-bacterial drugs.

Changes in health status are of course not always due to antecedent care. For many illnesses of young life, for example chicken-pox, there is no evidence that medical care influences outcome. For other diseases, whether or not a treatment is effective depends upon the choice of outcome measure. For example, appropriate prescription of analgesics may effectively relieve pain in patients terminally ill with cancer, but of course have no effect upon the progress of the disease itself. This is a trite example, but another will illustrate a finer point. A carefully controlled study showed that ACTH was effective in retrobulbar neuritis as judged by two outcome measures — an earlier relief of ocular pain, and an earlier return of central vision to test-type J1.[107] However, there was no evidence that ACTH influenced the *final* visual acuity achieved, nor is there evidence that ACTH influences the long-term natural history of multiple sclerosis.

The importance of defining outcome measures before starting clinical trials is now well recognised. The alternative — 'data dredging' — will show a difference significant at the 0.05 level once among twenty different univariate analyses. The definition of valid outcome measures when evaluating the quality of care is no less important. The difficulties are most apparent in chronic illness. In rheumatoid arthritis, for example, should the number of inflamed joints, joint erosions seen on X-ray, joint mobility, presence of pain, functional ability or level of erythrocyte sedimentation rate be taken as the outcome measure? The patient may be satisfied with temporary relief of pain and increased functional ability, but what if, in spite of these favourable effects, joint erosions are continuing under treatment A, but are suppressed by treatment B? And what if treatment B has more unpleasant side effects? Such questions can only be answered by very long-term clinical trials with standardised and pre-defined outcome measures.

It is surprising that after a century of scientific medicine we still do not really know the effects of therapeutic intervention on the long-term natural history of such common diseases as asthma and rheumatoid arthritis. The difficulties are compounded on occasion by direct contradiction between the results of health status indices and physiological measures of function. For example, Kaplan and colleagues[108] found that an exercise programme improved the health status of patients with chronic lung disease without any measurable benefit on lung function. Tattersfield[109] has found that, of two inhalers, children with asthma preferred the one that had less effect on improving peak flow.

A priority of any outcomes research therefore is the definition of agreed outcomes at different intervals after the onset of a disease. This statement pre-supposes an accurate classification of diseases, ie entities with a similar biology and a similar natural history without treatment — information that for most diseases is now simply not available, because they are not now studied without intervention of some type.

Disease-specific indices

Not only must the outcome be defined, but the methodology of measuring those outcomes must be agreed. For rheumatoid arthritis, for example, there are likely to be few worries now about measurement of the sedimentation rate, subject to adequate quality control in the laboratory, and this probably continues to be the best marker of *biological* disease activity.[110] But for measurement of *clinical* activity there remains considerable discussion. Should, for example, one count all inflamed joints, or should big ones like the knee joint count for more than the interphalangeal joints? Even when a disease-specific index is agreed by professional consensus — itself a noteworthy achievement — it must be remembered that the index is only an intermediate measure in one dimension. Swollen joints correlate to some extent with functional ability, but functional ability is influenced by age and prior disease activity rather than by current activity alone. Some examples of indices for other diseases are shown in Table 7.

Table 7. Examples of disease specific indices of health status.

Asthma — variation in peak expiratory flow

Rheumatoid arthritis — number of inflamed joints; goniometry

Depression — rating scales (Zung, Hamilton or Medical Outcomes Study[111]

Hypertension — level of systolic and diastolic pressure

Cancer — disease staging by tissue involvement

Coronary artery disease — successful angioplasty defined as 'less than 50% residual diameter stenosis; subsequent freedom for future angioplasty or coronary artery bypass graft surgery' [112]

Global measures of health status

Because of these difficulties, there has in the last fifteen years been a considerable interest in developing global measures of health status, functional status and the overall 'quality of life', which can be applied across different diseases.

Ware[113] suggests that the '. . . use of the quality of life nomenclature is likely to cause confusion because it is too encompassing. Jobs, housing, schools and the neighbourhood are not attributes of a person's health, and they are well outside the purviews of the health care system . . . . The goal of the health care system is to maximise the quality of life, namely health status.' Although sympathising with Ware's wish to limit to some extent those areas with which doctors should concern themselves, it must not be forgotten that poor housing and unemployment are both associated with illness. Leaving this point aside, however, it is useful to follow Ware's analysis of health into five principal concepts or dimensions — physical health, mental health, social functioning (adequacy of interpersonal relationships), role functioning (eg employment, school, housework) and perceived general health.

Very similar dimensions are reported by Segovia and colleagues after factor analysis of responses to a survey in Newfoundland.[114] The first factor in this study was related to disease (disability, chronic disease, worry about health); the second to happiness; the third to self-perceived health; the fourth and fifth to restriction of normal activities and social contacts.

There are a number of well accepted indices of health status which measure most of the dimensions specified by Ware, Segovia and colleagues.[113, 114] Two well known examples are the Nottingham Health Profile and the Sickness Impact Profile. As illustrations of the use of these scales, the Nottingham Health Profile has been used in an evaluation of the effectiveness of cardiac transplantation[115] and the Sickness Impact Profile in the quality of life of patients with breast cancer.[116] Many studies use combinations of these and other scales — for example one on the benefits of erythropoietin in patients on chronic haemodialysis.[116a]

A useful review of the problems of measuring quality of life in cancer is presented by Ebbs and colleagues.[117] A number of studies they cite report disparities between assessments made by doctors, nurses, the patient and his relatives. Slevin and colleagues concluded that 'a reliable and consistent method of measuring quality of life in cancer patients . . . must come from patients themselves, and not doctors and nurses.'[118]

Other general and disease-specific indices of health status are reviewed by Kind,[119] in a volume edited by Teeling-Smith,[120] and by a number of authors in a recent supplement to Medical Care.[121] Many of the available indices are related to physical function, for example, the Barthel index[122] and various modifications to the original Activities of Daily Living Scale of Katz (eg 123). As Ware[113] points out, too many of the available measures concentrate on negative aspects of health, and do not extend into the positive aspects of well-being and vitality.

Stewart, Ware and colleagues[124] point out that, to be clinically useful, measures of functional status of chronic conditions should be comprehensive in terms of the outcomes that are important to patients and be easy to administer. Scores should distinguish patients with chronic conditions from others with no chronic condition, and scores on each health component should correspond to specific features of the chronic condition. Within each condition, scores should vary for patients whose conditions differ in severity at a point in and over time. Finally, measures should be sensitive to the beneficial or harmful effects of treatment over time. Ware and colleagues have had considerable success[111, 124, 125] in using measures in relation to the first four of the points they propose. For eight chronic conditions such as angina, chronic back pain, depression and diabetes mellitus they were able to show that the measures they employed detected deviations from the scores of the general population without one of the conditions, although for the case of hypertension the only dimension in which deviation occurred was for self-rated perceptions of health. The profiles of deviations for different dimensions of functional status for four chronic conditions are illustrated in Fig. 3.

The scores obtained on sub-sections of measures such as the Medical Outcomes Study Short-Form General Health survey, employed by Ware's group,[111, 124, 125] the Nottingham Health Profile and the Sickness Impact Profile cannot be summed to provide a global one-figure measure of health as the scores represent different dimensions of health. My colleague Charles Warlow has pointed out that it would be no more meaningful to add up the results of a plasma electrolyte screen — say the sodium, potassium and urea levels — to obtain an 'electrolyte score'. There are practical as well as theoretical reasons for refusing to aggregate multi-dimensional scores. For example, in one study of the effectiveness of anti-hypertensive therapy on the quality of life, patients treated with captotril, methyldopa and propranolol had similar scores for disturbance of sleep and social participation, but those taking captotril scored significantly higher on measures of well-being and work performance. Those taking propranolol showed more evidence of sexual dysfunction.[126] An adverse effect that may be important to the quality of life of one person will be unimportant to another.

In spite of the multi-dimensionality of health, there have been continuing attempts to obtain some meaningful measure of health

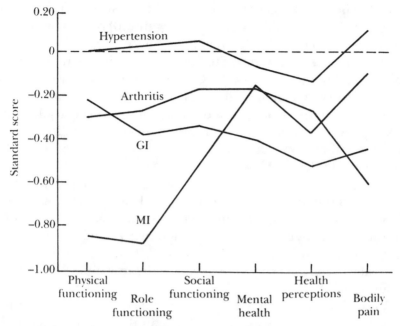

Fig. 3. *Health profiles for patients with four conditions (chronic gastro-intestinal disorder (GI), myocardial infarction (MI), arthritis and hypertension.* The dotted line is the standardised zero score for patients with no chronic conditions, obtained by setting the mean for each health measure on the Medical Outcomes Study Short-Form General Health Survey. Each chronic condition has a different and characteristic profile. Reproduced with kind permission from Stewart *et al.*[125]

status in a single figure, usually constrained between 1 (perfect health) and 0 (death). The best known are the Torrance time trade-off,[127, 127a, 128] a derivative of the standard gamble technique,[129] also used by Torrance, and the distress/disability matrices described by Rosser[130] now being improved as an Index of Health Related Quality of Life.[131] These have been reviewed in depth elsewhere (eg ref 120, 127–129), but a brief description is given here.

A 'single-figure' measure of quality of life is provided by the time trade-off technique of Torrance.[127, 127a, 128] Subjects are asked to judge how many years in a state of full health are equivalent to a given number of years in a described state of poor health. The ratio between the number of years is the utility, varying between 0 and 1, which can be considered as a value of the described health state to an individual, a summary figure from many dimensions. For examples, quoted by Torrance,[127] patients with kidney transplants judged their state to have a utility of 0.84; those who were anxious, depressed and lonely much of the time were judged to have a utility of 0.45. The use of the Torrance time trade-off technique for evaluating the different utilities of patients with different breast cancer scenarios is described by Buxton and Ashby.[128]

The Torrance time trade-off technique is a variant of the standard gamble technique, reviewed by Capewell.[129] Subjects are asked to choose between a gamble with a desirable outcome (eg restoration to health) with risk p, and a less desirable outcome (eg death), with risk $1-p$, and a certain option of intermediate desirability (eg survival with disability). The stated probabilities are varied until the subject is indifferent between the gamble and the certainty. The probability at the point of indifference can be used as a weight assigned to the intermediate health state. However, Hellinger[67] has shown that there is a significant variation in the risk attitudes among individuals for any given value, and a significant variability in the risk attitudes of a given individual towards different gambles. People generally become more averse to risk as the probability of death in a gamble increases.

Rosser and Watts[130] asked doctors to consider what information they used to assess the severity of illness in their patients, ignoring future prognosis. From their information eight descriptive statements emerged, for example, 'confined to chair or to wheelchair or able to move around in the home only with support from an assistant.' Distress was classified in four levels 'none', to 'severe'. Valuations (utilities) were then placed upon the resulting health states (eg 'confined to bed, mild distress'), by psychometric scaling using judges with different experiences of illness, including patients, doctors and nurses. The principal impact of the utilities derived from Rosser's work has been their use in the calculation of Quality Adjusted Life Years (QALYs).[131, 132]

The relationship between quality and quantity of life is illustrated in Fig. 4.[127] The quantity of life is the number of years from birth to death; the quality of life varies over time. The area under the graph is the number of undiscounted quality-adjusted life years (QALYs). A reasonable aim for medicine is to increase the area under the graph, either by 'ironing out' the dips in quality of life due to illness, or in prolonging life, or both. In an ideal life, the graph runs horizontally from birth, to dip down vertically at death.

Fries and colleagues[133] have pointed out that medical interventions, including promoting health, may compress morbidity, and extend active life expectancy (Fig. 5). He points out that some measure of increase in 'active life expectancy' should be used as an outcome measure. The same concept could — some would say 'should' — be used as a population outcome measure. Leaf writes 'Good

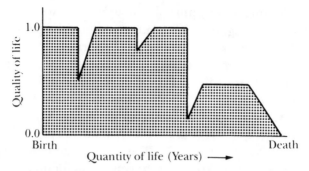

Fig. 4. *The relationship between quality and quantity of life.* The shaded area under the graph can be considered to represent the number of undiscounted quality-adjusted life years (QALYs). Re-drawn with kind permission from Torrance.[127]

health is much harder to define than duration of life, but it is a realistic goal for a health care system, and carries with it, as a likely bonus, the optimisation of the life span of each of us.' Establishing criteria on this basis would focus medical and public attention on the measures that are likely to promote optimal health, and on which measures must remain the responsibility of the individual and which that of the medical care system.[134]

For calculating the value of a treatment, some sort of notional dis-

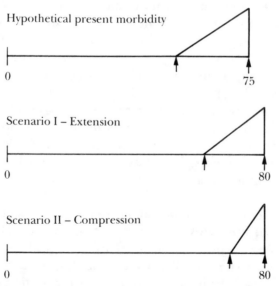

Fig. 5. *Morbidity towards the end of life.* This is represented by the triangles. It is perhaps more important to compress morbidity (scenario II) than to extend life (scenario I). Re-drawn with kind permission from Fries *et al.*[133]

counting of the future is required. The method is well explained by Donaldson and colleagues.[135] Without treatment, the patient survives *N1* years with health status (utility) *Q1* (derived from the Rosser matrix). With treatment, the patient survives *N2* years with health status *Q2*. The present value of the future years of life expectancy-can be computed at, say, a 5% discount to present values of *disc. N1* and *disc. N2*. The gain in quality-adjusted life years (QALYs) is then $(Q2 \times disc. N2) - (Q1 \times disc. N1)$. Williams presented a 'league table' of cost per QALY gained.[132] Kidney transplantation, for example, cost £3,000 per QALY, but hospital haemodialysis £14,000. However, Rosser has stressed the superficiality of such league tables.[131] Before utilities are used for judgements about cost-effectiveness, the concepts of equity and justice need to be introduced, or else few resources will be allocated to the elderly or handicapped. As Klein writes: 'There are many kinds of rationality, of which the economic variety is only one.'[136]

Some measurement of change in health status that can be linked to antecedent medical care would clearly be of high value in any medical unit, because without objective evidence of benefit there are no grounds for continuing our efforts. There are, however, a vast number of difficulties to be resolved. The first point is, whose valuations of health status should we use — the valuations of the general population, of doctors and nurses, or the valuations of the patients themselves?[118] The valuations are treated as static, whereas they may well shift as a result of experience of illness. In relation to cancer, Morris and colleagues[137] have written that as the disease progresses 'life takes on a new shape: it narrows, sometimes to a single room; work and running a household are no longer part of it. Friends and family are seen in a new way. Values change. What was once important may seem insignificant, while things once ignored have a great weight'. Furthermore, measurements of utility cannot readily be compared across different health programmes. For example, the utility for being anxious, depressed and lonely much of the time is similar to the utility of being blind or deaf or dumb,[127] which has little face validity.

Probably the most important barrier to the incorporation of measures of health status into everyday practice is the sheer impracticality of using the more sensitive measures of health status. Nelson and Berwick[138] write that 'We suspect that brevity, ease of administration (preferably by patients, perhaps during waiting room time), ease of scoring and simplicity of interpretation will be non-negotiable requirements for any instrument with a chance of achieving widespread use in stressed office settings.' The same restrictions will surely apply in routine hospital use.

Although measures of health status are able to distinguish between patients with different impairments, disabilities and handicaps,[125, 139] few measurement instruments are sufficiently sensitive to track changes in health status in individual patients. The principal benefit of measures of health status at present lies in defining need. For example, Williams and colleagues[140] found in a geriatric programme in New York State that the percentage of patients with appropriate placement was increased from 60% to 84% by the use of assessment measures. In a recent study, Lewis and colleagues[141] showed that dependence in performance of activities of daily living on admission to a nursing home was a powerful negative predictor of the probability of being able to return home, but so were even simpler measures — incontinence on admission, and the patient being a readmission rather than a first admission. Experienced physicians predict with fair accuracy which patients will do well, and which will do badly. The head-shaking that goes on over the coffee in sister's room presumably reflects the unconscious assessment of comparatively simple clinical variables and their relation to probable outcome that are more formally dissected in scales of functional status.

The recent White Paper,[1] probably influenced by such studies, requires all family doctors to make an annual functional assessment of all patients on their lists aged over 75 — but gives no guidance as to how this should be done. Here, surely, is a splendid opportunity for the National Health Service to gather information nationwide about our elderly population, by using nationally accepted standard measures of functional status.

Other points about measures of health status

Although 'quality of life' is usually thought of as a measure of outcome after medical intervention, it should be remembered that good quality process of care may help maintain a good quality of life during treatment, and this in turn increases the chances of a patient completing his treatment. Furthermore, the maintenance of a good quality of life may be a process measure influencing outcome. There is good evidence from some cancer trials that survival may be prolonged if the patient is encouraged to live as fully as possible, and work at communication with family and doctor.[142] Other evidence shows that impaired quality of life is a risk factor for cardiovascular disease.[143]

Measures of current health status can also be used to predict out-

come. Measures may again be disease specific — for example, relating to head injury,[144] or to abdominal aneurysm,[145] or more
general, as in the Glasgow coma scale.

The Medical Outcomes Study

Data is now emerging from the Medical Outcomes Study. This study
is a major initiative by Ware, Greenfield and associates [23, 124, 125, 146] to
understand how specific components of the system of delivery of
health care affect the outcomes of care by developing more practical
tools for monitoring patient outcomes, and by relating variations in
outcome to differences in the system from which the patient receives
care, and in the differences in clinicians' styles of practice. The study
is following the progress of patients with hypertension, diabetes,
coronary artery disease and depression, and undertaking cross-
sectional studies of these and other conditions. Stewart and
colleagues[125] have recently reported the variations in health profiles
for the four conditions. Preliminary evidence suggests that the measures are sufficiently sensitive to detect variations in disease severity,
and variations over time due to progression of the underlying
disease, or the effects of treatment.

Outcomes, effectiveness and costs

This publication is about the quality of care rather than cost, but
interested readers can refer to Weinstein and Stason,[135] Klein,[136]
Drummond[147] and Eisenberg[148] for a discussion of the measurement of cost-effectiveness and cost-benefit. The Oregon State
Government is the first to have moved towards the use of studies of
cost-effectiveness when allocating funds for different types of health
care. A Health Services Commission has been established to recommend 'a prioritised list of health services ranging from the most
important to the least important, based on the positive effects each
service has on the entire population, not just on a portion of it.'
Preliminary ratings suggest that the Commission will rank highly
family planning, antenatal and obstetric care, childhood immunisation and the treatment of acute illness. Speech therapy, infertility services, and plastic surgery all rate low.[149] Although this innovative
approach has provoked much heart searching, physicians must, as
Welch has said, be prepared to ask themselves some hard questions
relating to the trade-off between health care and other social goods.
'Are we sure that annual mammography is more important than a
Head-Start program?' 'Is one liver transplantation worth the price of
housing for four families?'[149]

At a more clinical level, one measure of outcome that physicians find intuitively useful is the number of patients that need to be treated to prevent one adverse event, such as a stroke or death. For example, the MRC trial of mild hypertension,[150] showed no reduction in mortality from all causes, but there was a significant reduction in the risk of stroke. However, it has been calculated that one would need to treat 31 patients with mild hypertension (<109 mmHg) for 20 years, in order to prevent one stroke,[151] a simple calculation which puts the benefits in perspective and against which the adverse effects of treatment can be placed.

This measure — the number of patients with a given disorder that a physician must treat in order to protect one of them from the disorder's potential consequences — has been calculated for a number of conditions and outcomes by Laupacis and colleagues[152] (Table 8). Mathematically, the number is equivalent to the reciprocal of the absolute reduction in risk — the difference in event rates between control and treatment groups, the data being obtained from randomised clinical trials. Laupacis and colleagues discuss how other measures of risk such as the relative risk reduction and odds ratio are relatively insensitive to differences in the magnitude of risk

Table 8. Number of patients that need to be treated to avoid outcomes.

	Condition	Outcome
1. Hypertension — (diastolic BP 90–114 mmHg)	Death, stroke, M.I.	
a. no target organ damage		17, for three years
b. with target organ damage		7, for three years
2. Stable angina, left main stem coronary disease: surgery	Death	6, by surgery
3. Transient ischaemic attack: aspirin	Death, stroke	6, for five years
4. Immunisation with hepatitis B vaccine:	Hepatitis	
general population		200
homosexual population		8
5. Breast cancer: screening of women aged 50–74	Death due to breast cancer	1592, for seven years

Data from Laupacis, Sackett and Roberts, 1988.[152]

of sub-groups without therapy. Table 8 helps place in perspective the value of treatments shown by randomised clinical trials to be undoubtedly efficacious.

Costs and quality

There was concern that the introduction of the Medicare prospective payment system linked to Diagnosis Related Groups in 1983 might influence the quality of care by limiting hospital expenditures. Certainly, there was thought that patients might be discharged 'quicker and sicker'.[153] Schramm and Gabel[154] review such information as there is. There were prominent changes in structure — accelerated rates of closure of hospitals, particularly of rural hospitals. Between 1983 and 1987, 45,000 hospital beds were removed from service, and full-time equivalent hospital employees declined by nearly 114,000. There were also changes in process; for example, the average length of stay declined by 9% in the first year of the programme. There was an enormous shift to the largely uncontrolled outpatient sector; 40% of hospital operations were performed in outpatient settings in 1986 as compared with 16% in 1980. Such shifts of care to different budgets may be compared to UK hospital practice since the introduction of district budgetary cash limits. Many physicians were asked to limit the prescription of drugs at discharge to no more than 7–14 days supply, thereby effectively shifting the costs of longer-term medication to family practitioner budgets.

As to outcome, in one study of a specific problem — fractured neck of femur — Fitzgerald and colleagues[155] found that after the change in method of Medicare reimbursement, patients with fractured hips received fewer physical therapy sessions as inpatients, were discharged sooner, and were significantly more impaired at discharge. The proportion of patients who could walk to any degree before discharge declined from 56 to 40% ($p < 0.04$). Patients were nearly four times more likely to be still in a nursing home one year after discharge.

Sager and colleagues[156] showed that although the proportion of deaths occurring in hospital declined between 1982 (65.1% of all deaths of Medicare enrollees) and 1985 (62.1%), this decline was largely balanced by an increase in the proportion of deaths occurring in nursing homes (from 18.9% to 20.8%). The figures suggest that patients were more frequently discharged to nursing homes for terminal care after the introduction of the prospective payment system. Although such care may be appropriate, Sager and colleagues[156] were concerned that not all nursing homes can be adequate substitutes for hospital services. Such concerns are reminiscent of those currently expressed in the UK[157] about the likely effects of the National Health Service and Community Care Bill upon after-care following procedures contracted to be performed in health districts far from the patient's home.

Patient satisfaction

Patient satisfaction is an important dimension of the outcome of health care. Apart from the fact that the consumer who pays for the services has a right to satisfaction, there are issues of health; a satisfied patient is more likely to follow appropriate medical advice. However, it must be remembered that one can have a satisfied patient who has had inappropriate investigation, incorrect diagnosis, inappropriate therapy and a less favourable outcome than could have occurred with treatment of better quality.

Just as the quality of medical care has several dimensions, of which patient satisfaction is one, so does satisfaction itself.[158] Patients can be satisfied or dissatisfied with accessibility of care, the technical aspects of care, interpersonal relationships with nurses and doctors, continuity of care, organisation of care, clarity of information received and the hotel services of the hospital or surroundings in outpatient clinics.

Methods of measuring patient satisfaction

One simple measure of patient dissatisfaction is to record the number and variety of complaints, which health districts in the UK have to record and to which they have to respond.[159] Repeated complaints about the same personnel or administrative function, such as a waiting list, call attention to areas that clearly require urgent attention. Isolated complaints, however, also have the virtue of indicating areas of organisational practice that no health professional had perceived to be a problem until the patient pointed it out.

A number of hospitals have published details of complaints received (eg 160), and references to a number of wider surveys are available in a literature review.[161] Inpatients most frequently complain about the amount of information received and relationships with doctors. Outpatients complain more about waiting times and other administrative problems. A bad institution may have few complaints simply because it makes it difficult for patients to complain. Indeed it has been shown that there is a positive correlation between the number of complaints (proxy for ease of making complaints) and patient satisfaction within the same institution. Patients may have the attitude (possibly justified) that it is 'no use complaining'. A friendly and reliable system of collecting complaints, and codifying them is a necessary prerequisite. There are certainly no reasons for believing that if there are no complaints then everything is going well. As Cryns and colleagues write[162] 'The antithesis of satisfaction is probably apathy or silent defection . . . Expressing dissatisfaction or complaining constitutes an involvement that is fundamentally different from being either satisfied or passively dissatisfied.' Because of this, it is right to explore actively patient satisfaction.

One way of trying to do this is by means of questionnaires which are either given to the patient on the ward, or mailed to him or her shortly after discharge. Although considerable time and effort has been devoted to devising such questionnaires, they often are in a similar simplistic form to those encountered in units of hotel chains aspiring to status, in which enquiry is made about satisfaction with reception, porterage and room service. Developing reliable questionnaires takes much time, as illustrated by the painstaking work of Ware and colleagues (eg 163). There is also the problem of validating them. Do the questionnaires actually measure what they set out to do? Fitzpatrick[164] has pointed out some of the difficulties in validating them. It is hard to conceive of ways of checking whether answers given to questionnaires reflect respondents' true views. However, he cites a number of studies which provide 'construct validity' — the extent to which relationships between measures conform to theoretical predictions. For example, Stiles and colleagues[165] showed that patients' satisfaction with their consultations in an outpatient clinic was related to the manner in which the doctor communicated, as measured independently.

There is the further difficulty that the responses vary according to how the questionnaire is administered. There is a bias if questionnaires are mailed, as those who are very satisfied or very dissatisfied may be presumed to be more likely to respond. On the other hand, if the questionnaire is to be completed before the patient leaves the ward or other care setting, it may be presumed that he is less likely to give unfavourable responses in order to avoid making 'enemies' among staff. Other biases include the fact that the sicker patients are too sick to respond to the questionnaire, and patients waiting for care — potentially dissatisfied — are not offered the opportunity to express this.

In spite of much effort to improve discrimination, 75% of all patients profess themselves as satisfied or very satisfied, so that assessment is working on a small margin, confused by natural variation.

With such high levels of satisfaction, it is difficult to have complete confidence in correlation between items as a measure of reliability. Satisfaction is not normally distributed, so the statistical handling of the results is not easy. Vast volumes of data can be produced, which requires input to a computer, although optically readable forms minimise this. Further criticisms of one questionnaire recently introduced in the UK[166] can be found in papers by Carr-Hill and colleagues.[167, 168]

Another way of measuring patient satisfaction is by means of an in-depth tape recorded non-schedule structured interview, which allows the respondent to voice in an open-ended fashion his feelings about the quality of his care (eg 169). This is probably the best way of exploring in depth patient satisfaction about a specific area of service or care, but it is expensive in terms of the time taken to interview, devise rating scales, and subsequently rate the tapes.

In general, the most convincing studies in satisfaction research are those in which particular issues are explored in relation to a particular client group or service by tape-recorded interviews in depth. From such interviews can be generated ideas for exploration by less expensive questionnaire techniques.[170]

Results of studies of patient satisfaction

Theoretical and practical exploration of patient satisfaction has identified a number of dimensions that are common to many clinical situations[163] — satisfaction about communication of information, personal manner of doctor or nurse (friendliness, concern), technical competence (thoroughness, accuracy), accessibility/convenience, (easy to get seen), outcome (getting better), continuity (same doctor at each visit) and physical environment (clean, pleasant), financial arrangements (eg insurance cover).

We cannot question the validity of patients' ratings of interpersonal aspects of care, as the consumer's viewpoint is the criterion.[171] Statements about accessibility and continuity are also fairly readily defined. What has taxed researchers is whether patients can distinguish technical care of good or bad quality, and thereby be satisfied or dissatisfied. There is some evidence, at least for common conditions that they can. Subjects were asked by Ware and colleagues to view videotapes of simulated consultations in which the content relating to necessary and sufficient physical history and examination was manipulated, whilst interpersonal attributes such as courtesy were held constant. The viewers rated more highly those consultations thought to be technically better by physicians (for references, see review, 171). However, there is a danger that patients may be seduced by quantity of technical process. Sox and colleagues studied middle-aged men with chest pain who had been determined on clinical grounds not to require investigations for myocardial infarction. Patients who were then randomly assigned to receive unnecessary tests (electrocardiogram and creatine phosphokinase) evaluated their care as better than did those who were not investigated.[172] However, this finding may reflect the particular culture in which this study was done — the USA. In the UK, my study with Fitzpatrick of patients with headache not due to structural disease showed that whether or not a patient was investigated was not a feature associated with patient dissatisfaction.[169] In this study, 34% of headache patients were dissatisfied with some aspect of their consultations, many statements centering on the fact that the neurologist was considered to have been 'too superficial and routine' in going through their histories, and did not sufficiently explore the meaning to them of the headaches, and how the headaches influenced their lives.

Again, this discouragingly high level of dissatisfaction may be an attribute of the particular service studied. In other circumstances, doctors feel that they have done less well in consultations than the patients say they have. Rashid and colleagues[173] aimed to identify those aspects of a consultation in which patients or doctors agreed or disagreed that an acceptable level of care had been provided. Table 9 illustrates two of the areas of disagreement, in both of which

Table 9. Agreement between doctors and patients about some aspects of the acceptibility of care.

	Patient Yes/ Doctor Yes (%)	Patient No/ Doctor Yes (%)	Patient Yes/ Doctor No (%)	Patient No/ Doctor No (%)
Did the doctor give the patient an opportunity to ask any necessary questions? ($n = 222$)	70	3	25	2
Did the patient feel it was worth coming to the consultation overall? ($n = 220$)	81	2	16	<1

Data from Rashid *et al.* [173]

the doctor felt that they had done significantly worse than the patients thought they had.

There are other areas of disagreement. Doctors, nurses, administrators and patients have been asked to rank aspects of care that they consider to be most important to patients — and there is little agreement between the rankings.[174]

Thompson asked hospital patients in the United Kingdom whether they would be willing to return to the same hospital if necessary. Overall, 60% said that they were very happy to return, 33% were indifferent, and 7% indicated that they would prefer to go elsewhere. Thompson isolated a number of dimensions of satisfaction/dissatisfaction, and found that the most important determinant of the response to this question was nursing care (9% of the variance), food and physical facilities (7%), and medical care and information (5%).[175]

The following generalisations may be made from published studies. Satisfaction declines as the hospital visit recedes in time. Patients complain more about organisational problems than their relatives. Families of patients complain more about technical aspects of health care and nursing care than do patients themselves. It could be argued that the focus should be on the patient, as the consumer, and not on the family, but members of the family are of course potential consumers.

There are other points of interest. A number of studies show that age, sex and socio-economic group do not correlate with patient satisfaction. Most but not all studies suggest that the severity and degree of evolution of illness do not correlate with patient satisfaction.

Virtually all those who have worked on patient satisfaction conclude that it is necessary to focus enquiry on one particular client group or clinic or service, as points of particular dissatisfaction are often peculiar to that group. It has already been mentioned that the concerns of inpatients and outpatients are different, and, as a further example, satisfaction about personal financial arrangements is not relevant to the NHS. All that questionnaires can do is to provide a system of alerting clinicians and managers to problems the solution of which will usually require a focused study.

Different perspectives on quality

A recent study from general practice has forcefully indicated how individuals have different priorities from those which their government thinks they ought to have. Smith and Armstrong[183] found that patients ranked most highly having a doctor who listens, having a doctor who sorts out problems, and usually seeing the same doctor, all criteria generated through preliminary interviews with another group of patients. The three criteria least highly valued were health education, being able to change doctor easily, and well decorated and convenient premises, all amongst criteria of good practice originated by the government. Of other government criteria, only regular screening for breast and cervical cancer, and regular health checks for adults (of dubious effectiveness, see p. 61) found widespread support among patients. Smith and Armstrong conclude that there seems to be limits to both consumer sovereignty and professional authority in good practice.

5 | Quality in screening and health promotion

The framework of this paper has so far discussed quality for patient care. But of importance also is a brief discussion of health promotion and screening. Many of the same issues apply: for example, screening has to be relevant to the population, but it must be remembered that there is no point in finding disease unless effective treatment can be offered. In addition, a whole additional range of quality issues apply, relating to the achievement of low false positive and false negative rates, the psychological costs to the patient of screening[176] and the recall systems. Principal among these issues is the effectiveness as a whole of screening programs.

A recent review by Oboler and LaForce[177] reports that 'for the asymptomatic, non-pregnant adult of any age, no evidence supports the need for a complete physical examination as traditionally defined'. Their review does, however, go on to marshall evidence for the efficacy of three screening procedures — the measurement of blood pressure every two years; examination of the breasts of women aged more than 40 years; a pelvic examination and a Papanicolaou smear for sexually active women every three years after two initial negative tests at intervals of one year. There is no evidence that screening for lung cancer is effective.[178] Less convincing evidence suggests that a few other procedures such as a palpation of the abdomen of men aged over 60 on an annual basis in order to exclude abdominal aneurysms, are prudent. This review[177] is important as it allows the development of one methodology for assessing the quality of care in primary practice. This is recognised by the Government in the National Health Service and Community Care Bill which will authorise increments in pay to general practitioners if defined targets for cervical smears are achieved.

The whole issue of the appropriateness, quality and effectiveness of screening programs is considered in a monograph by Holland,[179] so will not be further considered here. Health promotional programs also lie outside the principal focus of this book, and the criteria used for assessing their quality must be different, and perhaps more related to the field of advertising, with the exception of their effectiveness and efficiency. Warner[180] reports that there is good information on the economics of intervention policies in only two areas of health promotion — stopping smoking, and control of hypertension. For other areas, such as the cost-effectiveness of programmes for the prevention of back injury, there is virtually no information.[181] The impact of campaigns to reduce smoking is hard to distinguish from other social changes.[182]

6 | Some examples of evaluation of the effectiveness of care and of medical audit

The following examples are some of many that could have been used to illustrate the principles described in this book.

The management of chest pain

Emerson and colleagues reviewed the management of 604 patients with chest pain attending an accident and emergency department.[184] Expert assessors, who knew the results of any subsequent investigations, judged that 119 should have been admitted to the coronary care unit, and of these 14 (11.8%) were judged to have been sent home in error, most commonly because of errors in interpreting the electrocardiogram (ECG). Of the 485 patients whom the assessors judged should not have been admitted, 32 (6.6%) were advised admission unnecessarily, according to the assessors. The median waiting time for those eventually admitted to the coronary care unit was 78 minutes.

In another study, Sharkey and colleagues analysed the time delays before the administration of lytic therapy to patients with a myocardial infarction.[185] After arrival in the emergency department, patients waited for an average of 20 minutes before the first ECG, and a further 70 minutes before lytic therapy began. Delays were shorter if lytic therapy was given in the emergency department rather than in the coronary care unit, and the authors suggest this as a routine.

Problems with pacing

An audit of problems arising with the insertion of temporary pacing showed a high proportion of failures to pace and significant rates of infection when the pacemaker was inserted at a general hospital rather than a cardiac centre.[186]

Ambulance transfer of patients

Of 200 consecutive patients comatose after head injury in West Scotland, only 42% were transported to a neurosurgical unit with an endotracheal tube in place, and half of these had been transported in the supine position, at risk from inhalation.[186a] Another paper from West Scotland audited the support requirements in transport of 378 critically ill patients.[186b]

Non-attendance of patients

An audit of why some patients called for ENT operations did not have their operations showed that the rate of non-attendance by patients was 14.6%.[187] Although an upper respiratory tract infection was the most frequent reason for non-attendance, the second most frequent reason for the operation not being done was that a consultant review found the planned operation to be unnecessary. Such patients had often been put on the waiting list by doctors in training, suggesting that a more active involvement of consultants in out-patient clinics was required.

Use of birth centres

Free standing birth centres offer a safe and acceptable alternative to hospital confinement for selected pregnant women, particularly those who had previously had children, and such care leads to relatively few Caesarian sections.[188]

Use of beds

Elective cardiac catheterisation can safely be undertaken as an out-patient procedure with complication rates not significantly different from those catheterised as an inpatient. However, 12% of those catheterised as outpatients did require admission to hospital because of complications of catheterisation.[189]

Patients may be admitted to or retained in hospital inappropriately. An audit of 847 admissions to hospital in Oxford showed that for only 38% of bed days were patients considered to have medical, nursing or life support reasons for requiring a bed.[57] The authors suggest that an increased frequency of consultant ward rounds or delegating discharge decisions to others might reduce the inappropriate use of beds. Similar inappropriate use has been reported for the use of paediatric beds.[55]

Closure of beds in a district hospital increases the number of days in a year in which the hospital is full and closed to further admissions from general practitioners, and is associated with an increase in the proportion of very elderly patients admitted, and in the proportion of self-referred patients.[189a]

Admitting elderly patients to hospital to give temporary relief to their carers is not associated with increased mortality. [189b]

Use of time

Short as opposed to long general practitioner consultations result in less attention being paid to psychosocial issues that the doctor recognises as relevant. When psychosocial problems were dealt with, antibiotic prescribing decreased.[190]

Use of physical therapy

No difference in outcome was achieved in a randomised controlled trial of physical therapy for spastic diplegia.[191] Fewer patients with acute neck sprains resulting from road traffic accidents had symptoms two years later if they had received advice on early mobilisation than those who received manipulative physiotherapy or advice to rest.[192]

Use of appliances

Of 82 patients prescribed surgical footwear, 66 continued to wear them after two years, but half of these had difficulty in putting on their shoes, a problem that could have been overcome in many instances by the use of Velcro fasteners.[193]

Use of X-rays

Skull X-rays after trauma

Very large numbers of skull X-rays are carried out on patients attending Accident and Emergency Departments after head injury. Masters and colleagues[194] defined a low risk-group in whom X-ray was not indicated. The definition was then validated by an audit of more than 7,000 patients. The risk of missing intracranial sequelae because an occult skull fracture is not diagnosed in a low-risk patient is very small — it is 95% likely to be no higher than 3 per 10,000 ($p < 0.0003$).

X-rays of the cervical spine

An anterior-posterior radiograph of the cervical spine contributes virtually no further information than that derived from a lateral film in patients with cervical pain not due to trauma, unless there is clinical suspicion of a cervical rib.[195] The prevalence of spondylotic changes in those referred for cervical spinal X-rays is no higher than in a control group, referred for barium meal examinations.[196]

Chest X-rays

Hubbell and colleagues[197] have reviewed the impact of routine admission chest X-rays upon patient care. Films were ordered for 294 (60%) of the 491 patients studied. Abnormalities were noted in 106 (36%) of these 294 patients. However, the findings were previously known, chronic, and stable in 86 patients. They were new in only 20, and treatment was changed as a result of these X-rays in only 12 of the patients. In only one of the patients would appropriate treatment probably have been omitted had the X-ray not been done.

Myelography

The area of the spinal canal specified for particular examination was clinically inappropriate in 11% of more than 300 patients submitted for myelography.[198]

Availability of X-rays in clinics

Bransby-Zachary and Sutherland[199] found that 141 of 420 patients attending an orthopaedic clinic in a major hospital in Glasgow had had previous X-rays arranged by their general practitioner. Only nine patients had X-ray films available when they attended the orthopaedic clinic. As 'radiography is an integral part of the orthopaedic examination', 125 of the 132 patients whose films were not available had their X-ray examination repeated. 'The (orthopaedic) specialist ordered most of the repeat examinations, so they can be assumed to be appropriate for effective patient management.' Although the authors plead for improved administrative arrangements, they give no evidence to support the statements in quotes.

Communication of X-ray results

All of a sample of 32 clinicians thought that radiologists should always tell patients immediately about the result of their X-ray if it was normal. Of 33 radiologists, 11 thought that this was only occasionally appropriate.[199a]

Use of biochemistry

Morgan[200] has shown that routine urine testing continues to be useful, leading to new diagnoses after investigation in 27 out of 5,886 patients (about 0.5%) attending a variety of outpatient clinics, most commonly diabetes mellitus. What he does not remark upon is that in a further 61 patients, abnormalities had been noted, but no further evaluation had been carried out. A literature review indicates that for patients under the age of 50, routine urine testing is a sufficient biochemical pre-operative screen, and that multiple analyses of serum are not necessary.[201] Further references are available.[201a]

Use of microbiology

Flanagan and colleagues have evaluated four screening tests for bacteriuria in elderly people[202] — visual appearance; microscopy; dipstick for nitrite, leucocyte esterase, protein and blood; dipstick for nitrite and organisms. A combination of visual appearance and dipstick testing for nitrite and leucocyte esterase gave a sensitivity of 96%, a specificity of 50%, a positive predictive value of 57% and a negative predictive value of 95%. If neither of these tests is positive, the urine can safely be discarded without microscopy or culture.

Effectiveness of treatment

Effective control of diabetes mellitus, as judged by a lower mean level of glycated haemoglobin measured at intervals over the previous six years, is associated with lesser degrees of retinopathy, even if the duration of the diabetes is taken into account.[203]

Patients with cancer and a single metastasis to the brain live longer and enjoy a better quality of life if the tumour is surgically removed, followed by radiotherapy, than if radiotherapy alone is given.[203a]

Significant reductions in serum lipid levels can be achieved in patients attending a lipid clinic, but target levels are achieved in only about 40% of patients.[203b]

Errors in medication

Raju and colleagues[204] found in a prospective study in neonatal and paediatric intensive care units that an error in medication arose in one per 6.8 admissions (14.7%). There was one iatrogenic injury per 33 admissions, and a tenth of these were potentially serious. The most frequent errors arose due to drugs being given at the wrong time, at the wrong rate, or in the wrong dose. Sixty per cent of the events were nursing errors. In another study, Beers and colleagues found that in 10% of emergency room visits at which medication was added, a new medication could potentially have caused an adverse interaction.[204a]

7 | The way forward

Brook and Kosecoff[8] have written:

> We have read hundreds of papers about quality of care. Most contain little or no data. Most proclaim the need for more and better data. Most make conclusions even where there are no data. Should they be read?

I am conscious that this review may fall into the same trap, but I do believe that from the preceding sections of this book, a physician, or a manager, can construct a 'shopping list' of topics for audit, and now make an impact on the quality of care in his or her own hospital or health district. There are so many problems crying out for evaluation that it is reasonable to say that it hardly matters *what* is audited, except that some attempt is made to measure in a meaningful way some dimension of quality of care, possibly picked from those illustrated in earlier chapters and in Table 10. It would seem sensible to concentrate on areas about which concern is already being expressed in the community or institution. These may be

Table 10. Examples of subjects suitable for prospective audit. (See also Table 6)

Use of skull X-rays in the Accident and Emergency Department
Accuracy of diagnostic coding
Waiting time for appointment in Outpatients
Waiting times for 'cold' surgery — eg herniorrhaphy, coronary bypass surgery, hip replacement, varicose veins
Proportion of results of investigations filed
Use of chest X-rays in patients under age 60
Appropriateness of Holter monitoring
Adequacy of anticoagulation
Interval between discharge and posting discharge summary
Repeat blood counts at intervals of less than two weeks
Use of hypnotic/psychotropic medication in the elderly
Urinary infections after catheterisation
New pressure sores
Inappropriate hospital days
Inappropriate investigation in defined conditions
Process of diabetic care
Inadequate follow-up of detected hypertension

simple problems such as accessibility (waiting times) for hip replacement, or a problem related to the speedy return of biochemical
results, or a problem as complex as a series of suicides in the
psychiatric unit. Useful guidelines as to the administrative structure
necessary to formalise audit are given by Shaw and Costain.[204b]

For reasons advanced on p. 25, I do not believe that large scale
audit of the written hospital record is a sufficiently sensitive and
inexpensive way of 'getting at' the quality of patient care. I must also
confess to a personal bias here. I do not believe that a good written
record encourages a good interpersonal relationship with the
patient. I have already quoted the patient who complained after a
consultation that 'he never even looked at me; he was too busy writing.' The notes of colleagues in other specialties who are rightly
sought after for their clinical expertise and humane care are often
frankly deficient when I see their patients on inpatient consultations. Very often mine are little better, and I find it easier to write
a coherent opinion away from the bed than to write a note during
the hurly-burly of taking a history. It is also not easy to write a sensible follow-up note that reflects all the changing problems in an
episode of illness, although problem-oriented medical records do
make this more straightforward.[204c] All notes must be sufficient to
allow continuity of care, particularly as the hours of work of hospital
doctors shorten and more doctors and nurses are involved in any
one episode of care.

What may be termed 'aggressive' record keeping has swept
through nursing in the UK and the USA. On entering a ward, a consultant is more likely to find his ward sister behind a desk rather than
by a bed. Wiener and Kayser-Jones have analysed nursing work in this
regard.[205] Their paper entitled 'Defensive work in nursing homes:
accountability gone amok' reviews how extensive record keeping
designed to protect the institution or individual encourages acceptance of care of low standard and diversion of attention from therapeutic work. Physicians would not wish undue attention to the
written record to distort their work in a similar way. Although many
of us in the UK believe our health service is bureaucratic, the
amount of paper-work involved in treating patients is minimal compared to the horrendous proliferation so wittily described by
Grumet in the USA,[206] where the physician has to struggle for reimbursement of his fees by a welter of third-party providers. The
changes proposed in the National Health Service and Community
Care Bill are likely to increase considerably the keeping of records
for financial reasons by UK doctors, who remain unconvinced that
they will be served by adequate information systems.

I must also confess to some unfashionable reservations about computers. For some reason, the concept of audit has in the UK become entangled with the provision of better information systems. It is true that a good computerised patient information system or a Departmental micro-computer may allow more accurate indicators of throughput, 'performance' and costs, but, with regard to quality, there are still grave difficulties about deciding what information can be entered into a computer that is a realistic measure of quality of care. It is also true that very large data bases, such as those maintained by Medicare and by the Commission on Professional and Hospital Activities, linked to PRO reviews of medical records, can determine associations between, for example, pre-operative clinical variables and post-operative mortality. As an example, Roper and colleagues[207] report that a history of congestive cardiac failure increases the risk after coronary bypass surgery by a factor of 1.9, but after angioplasty by a risk of 4.0, a difference not apparently accounted for by assigning higher risk patients to the less major procedure. However, such analyses still provide no information about the quality of care of individual patients.

Although I do not believe that better information systems will 'do' audit, there is no doubt that the collection and analysis of large volumes of data may throw into relief unexpected problems or variations in the process of practice or in outcomes of care.[208] A recent example is the largely unexpected finding that patients undergoing an open prostatectomy for benign hyperplasia had a lesser mortality than patients undergoing transurethral prostatectomy — a difference that remained even when corrections were made for associated medical conditions.[209] This is the value of large databases, but to attempt to *explain* such problems or variations usually requires an explicit research project.

Audit is rather easier in surgical than in medical practice, where outcomes are related to the event of the operation itself. Perioperative mortality, unplanned return to the operating theatre, removal of normal tissue and wound infection (if adequately defined) are variables that can fairly readily be gathered on to a simple database, on unit, district, regional or even national scale. For audit of physicianly care, there are a number of groups attempting to specify an effective data set for some common illnesses. However, none of the adverse outcomes of care listed in Table 6 can be used to monitor quality unless the measures are valid and sensitive and, most importantly, unless there are in place reliable systems for collecting information about adverse outcomes.

I believe a better approach is to mount a mini-research project on one or more of these possible indicators, with a defined method of data collection prospectively from a defined population. It will usually be necessary to assign a member of staff or an outside researcher to such a project. For example, a young physician in training could for a period of six months visit each ward in a hospital twice a day to record all infusions and transfusions, by whom they had been set up, and the rates of tissue infiltration and infection. He could audit the appropriateness of each transfusion by pre-determined criteria,[98] review the appropriateness of the infusions and the fluids used, and review the clarity with which instructions were given to the nursing staff. The fact that his intrusion on to the ward might improve the quality with which infusions are given during the course of his or her project is irrelevant, as the whole purpose of audit is educational.

Even with on-going improvement during the course of his project, the young doctor is likely to come up with recommendations to his institution that will improve the quality of this aspect of patient care. However, further, probably briefer, evaluations will need to be made from time to time to ensure that there has been no falling back to the old standards, and to ensure that improvements in technique and in equipment since the previous evaluation have been incorporated into the procedure. This is the audit 'cycle' as described by Shaw.[6] For such studies, health districts and regions should budget a significant sum each year out of their operational expenditure. Such locally generated autonomous audits are likely to be carried out with a greater level of enthusiasm and satisfaction than audits imposed centrally. Furthermore, the selection of topics is likely to be relevant to the immediate problems recognised locally.

Coles also has stressed that 'Audit should proceed from the particular to the general, and from concrete personal experience to abstract collective responsibility'.[210] It has to be recognised, however, that local hospital politics may get in the way of neutral assessment, and the projects may be carried out with different degrees of thoughtfulness. It is here that District and Regional Directors of Public Health in the UK can provide the epidemiological skills and degree of detachment from everyday clinical life that will allow successful audit studies. I firmly believe that such evaluations of quality are more appropriate projects for many young doctors training for a consultant post than more formal but often repetitive and unorganised biological research, the publication of which at present clogs much of the medical literature.

Doctors have always recognised that it is unjustified to carry out inappropriate and ineffective treatment; what is inappropriate and ineffective must therefore clearly be principal topics for research in the future, and physicians then educated about the results. In the USA, The Department of Health and Human Services, through the Health Care Financing Administration and the Public Health Service has decided 'to take an active role in improving the quality of medical information that guides medical practice',[207] and Ellwood[211] has written of the need to help 'patients, payers and providers make rational medical care-related choices based on better insight into the effect of these choices on the patient's life, choices that are likely to be informed by research directed towards appropriateness of investigations and procedures, and outcomes.'

Brook has stressed the potential value of practice guidelines, writing that there is a need for an 'institution' to develop and maintain-guidelines that are outcome based and outcome justified. As he writes, there is a danger that 'everybody is still off doing their own thing . . . such a process produces a low quality product.' Such an 'institution' must be nationally based, as the guidelines must reflect the different ways in which health care is delivered, the different cultural perspectives of the population (both patients and doctors), and the resources available. Guidelines produced in the US, although informative, may be of little use to the population of Bangladesh, who will have quite different priorities. Even between two culturally similar countries — the UK and the US — guidelines of appropriateness did not prove to be readily transferable.[53]

The Royal Colleges and their Faculties in the UK are well placed to act as 'institutions' of the type envisaged by Brook. The Research Unit of the Royal College of Physicians is undertaking an intensive programme of workshops in association with specialist societies at which such guidelines will be developed for a number of common medical conditions, following a lead given by the Clinical Efficacy Assessment Project of the American College of Physicians. Workshops have so far been held on the management of urinary infections in childhood, on the management of chronic neurological illness, and on various aspects of the care of elderly people. Others planned for the near future include the management of inflammatory arthropathies, of febrile convulsions and of asthma in adults. It is a particular feature of these workshops that members are asked to consider audit measures through which departures from guidelines can be detected.

Guidelines may guide physicians in appropriate practice, and an appropriate procedure is more likely to be effective in relieving symptoms, but unwanted outcomes may still occur. Wennberg's group[213, 214] has stressed the relatively high rate of unwanted outcomes after the commonly performed operation of prostatectomy.

Fifteen per cent of patients had episodes of acute retention due to blood clots, for more than half of whom catheterisation was required. Twenty per cent of patients reported a post-surgical infection, and for a third of these the infection lasted two or more weeks. Five per cent of patients lost their ability to have erections after surgery, and four per cent were incontinent. Wennberg and colleagues[213] stressed how patients with similar pre-operative symptoms such as frequency were bothered to a considerably different extent by their symptoms. They stress how the significance of the symptoms before the operation, and the significance of good and bad outcomes to the patient, must play a major role in the decision about whether 'watchful waiting' or surgery is the correct choice.[214] This, then, is another way forward: to inform the patient clearly and accurately of the probable outcomes of an intervention, and involve him more fully in decisions about his care.

There remains an urgent need for research into the methodology of the evaluation of health status. We can build upon the utility framework advanced by Torrance, Rosser and others (pp. 44–51), but it is necessary to explore further the reasons why a utility level is chosen, and to consider further the implications of the population chosen to rank different states of health. What are the components of ill-health that subjects find most distressing, and do their rankings change if ill-health is experienced? How can natural equity be linked in to rankings of utility and QALYs?[127a, 131, 215] What are the correlations between different ways of measuring quality of life? What are the best ways of measuring illness severity, so that this can be taken into account when judging outcome?

While such research is going forward, there would, I believe, be considerable benefit if physicians accepted that life is imperfect, and agreed to use a limited number of well-validated indices both of severity of illness and functional outcome, so that comparisons can be made with care delivered in different settings and different health districts. There would be considerable advantages also if the Department of Health recommended one of the many available patient satisfaction questionnaires, and districts standardised the method of administration. One of the advantages of a National Health Service should be the ability to collect large volumes of data on a national basis. In the USA, accurate documentation of diagnosis is required for Medicare reimbursement, and the resulting large data-base allows good opportunities for epidemiological research (eg 58, 208, 213, 214).

Although one way forward in medicine will continue to be through advances in biological science, and through randomised

controlled trials for studying the effectiveness of the possibilities
thrown up by scientific medicine, the evaluation of *clinical practice* by
such models requires that our objectives and our criteria for success
are unambiguous, and that what constitutes clinical practice can itself
be precisely specified. However, as Carr-Hill writes, it is precisely these
prerequisites that are challenged by sociological accounts of practice.[216] Leaving aside theoretical analyses of clinical work, we need to
incorporate methodologies from other sciences, particularly social
science, into our work.[217] If return to work is regarded as an outcome
of good medical management, we cannot ignore social factors such
as the state of the job-market, or the opportunity for modification to
work routines. What type of family structure or what dimensions of
housing give rise to greatest independence in old age? What are the
best social structures within hospitals that will allow change?

We also need to be much more explicit about defining the objectives of our care. For example, what are we trying to achieve by a routine follow-up hospital outpatient appointment for a patient with
chronic locomotor disability, due to rheumatological or neurological disease? Are the patient's symptoms and concerns appropri-
ately handled in this way, or would we do better to intervene only
when requested by the patient or his family doctor?

We also need to consider and research further into how to encourage changes in practice as a result of audit, an issue that is addressed
in few of the published studies about audit. Mitchell and Fowkes[218]
and Eisenberg[219] review the evidence that audit and feedback of the
results changes clinical practice, and they find a depressing lack of
evidence that this is so, particularly in regard to the ordering of investigations. Small changes in behaviour in the desired direction can be
obtained by active education at a personal level by a respected senior
colleague when feeding back the results. Most reports are of projects
of short duration, and there is as yet little evidence that any change
is long-standing, and not just a short-term response to a new initiative. The costs of feed-back programs are in themselves significant,
and may nullify the savings in costs achieved by the program.[219]
However, leaving the question of cost aside, we can be encouraged
by reports that rates of inappropriate Caesarian section can be
reduced, although Myers and Gleicher found that an individualised
approach[220] is much more successful than the dissemination of
good practice through guidelines.[45] Stafford,[220a] in the context of
Caesarian section, has reviewed the impact and feasibility of these
and other strategies for controlling rising rates of Caesarian section.
Alternative strategies include external review of practices, reform of
medical malpractice, modification of reimbursement of hospitals

or of obstetricians, education, including public dissemination of section rates, and peer evaluation. Some success has also been achieved with reducing requests for inappropriate radiological examinations.[221]

It may be that practice styles are fixed very early in a medical career. If so, it is of the utmost importance that undergraduate teaching hospitals take a robust attitude to encouraging appropriate investigation and treatment — an attitude in potential conflict with much of their work as tertiary referral centres, often undertaking intensive and invasive investigations. The changing cultural climate of medical practice — that to consider appropriateness and costs carefully is an essential part of practice — makes such teaching obligatory. There is some evidence from a very recent paper[221a] that such interventions are more effective than previously reported.

The medical profession in the UK has by and large welcomed the concept of medical audit, recognising it as a worthy extension of the concept of scientific medicine. There is, however, a general feeling that the Department of Health does not recognise the difficulty of using on an everyday basis measures of health status which have been developed for research purposes. Some physicians and surgeons believe that they are operating effectively, and that it is constraints on resources that limit the quality of their care. The arguments advanced in this review, particularly the wide regional variations in rates of referral and surgical operation and lengths of stay indicate that some resources can certainly be released for better patient care, but there are two areas in which there is almost universal professional belief that limited resources constrain quality. The first is in waiting times for elective surgery. We have in the UK the lowest number of trained surgeons per capita in the Western world. Secondly, salaries are so low that there are grave difficulties in recruiting and retaining medical records staff and secretaries. A surgeon might at present very reasonably say that 'I will reduce my waiting list and get the discharge summaries out on time if the district appoints a further consultant surgeon and gives us more theatre time and more secretarial help.' In short, the distinction must be made between an issue of quality related to the provider of health care and resource constraints. It is necessary that the Government recognises the strength of this feeling, and undertakes that resources released by, for example, more day care as opposed to inpatient surgery are channelled into tangible improvements elsewhere in the system.

Research should also continue into the value of commonly used procedures for which there is little evidence of effectiveness. An example is the widespread use of poorly validated physical methods of treatment such as ultrasound for backache and muscle strains. Continual research into the natural history of disorders, and its modification by treatment will allow more accurate probabilities of outcome on which clinical decision analysis can be based. Until such probabilities are widely available, groups of experienced clinicians, joined by consumers, should continue to construct guidelines of good management against which care can in future be audited. The funding of such research into effectiveness, which requires the definition and measurement of outcomes of medical intervention, should receive high priority from the Department of Health, as is planned from the Federal Government in the United States.[222]

8 | Conclusion

Relman[223] has written that we are now on the threshold of a third revolution in medical care. The first was the rapid expansion of scientific medicine and hospital technology, the second was the 'Revolt of the Payers — the Era of Cost Containment.' The third, he suggests, is the 'Era of Assessment and Accountability.' He writes that 'in order to provide a basis for decisions on the future funding and organisation of health care, we will have to know more about the variations in performance among institutions and medical practitioners and what these may mean. We will also need to know much more about the relative costs, safety and effectiveness of all the things physicians do or employ in the diagnosis, treatment and prevention of disease.' One of the central themes of the White Paper[1] is that we should be more aware of the costs of what we do, and that, as Sullivan writes '. . . a reasonable amount of competition and choice may offer (us) the best opportunity to preserve high quality care.'[224]

I concur with Donabedian's approach[9] that neutrality and detachment are needed in studies of quality. He writes 'More often one needs to ask "What goes on here?" rather than "What is wrong; and how can it be made better".' At all times it is necessary to understand the process of care first before evaluating quality. Berwick[40, 138] has stated that a priority is that an operational system must be agreed by all workers in a segment of a health care system, and the goals and characteristics of performance must be defined. He, and Laffel and Blumenthal[225] have both stressed the lessons that can be learned from experience gained from industrial quality management science, which recognises the complexity of many processes of production, and the need to focus on the process, rather than the individual worker, when striving to improve quality.[226]

Berwick has also stressed that respect for the health care worker must be re-established. Many doctors at present feel under siege by the community and politicians that do not comprehend the stresses of their work. Berwick stresses that quality is likely to improve further if all workers are already assumed to be doing their best, but will try even harder if better systems of care are introduced. When physicians and other health care workers, he writes, '. . . are caught in complex systems and performing complex tasks, of course clinicians make mistakes, these are unintentional, and the people involved cannot be frightened into doing better . . . they will be wasting their time in self defence instead of learning. '[93] This then is the root of this review — that medical audit and assuring medical care of good quality is an educational and not a punitive concept.

Finally, physicians must be more sensitive to the patient's perspective.[227] Physicians' accounts of their own illnesses often have as a central theme their stark realisation of their change in role, of what it is like to be a patient — the failure to relieve pain promptly, the waiting for the results of biopsies and the conflicting information given by different members of staff. But there are more subtle aspects to consider too, particularly in relation to outpatient practices. Patients do not come to doctors with clean slates upon which a diagnosis and management is imposed. Rather they have their own concepts of illness and explanations for their symptoms. Hunt and colleagues explored feelings about illness and diagnosis through extensive interviews and concluded that

> while it is rare that the medical diagnosis is rejected outright, it is almost always modified as it interacts with concepts the individual has assembled from a variety of sources as they try to make the explanation 'liveable'. Diagnosis must fit with the concepts and circumstances of patients' daily lives, or it will be reworked to accommodate them . . . The medical interaction is but one of many social constraints . . . The picture that emerges is one of a continuing process in which (the patient's) tentative ideas are built up and elaborated as they are exposed to the exigencies of everyday life.[227]

The individuality of life and response to illness is something that a doctor must always recognise; if he does, there will be few complaints about the quality of his care.

References

1 *Working for patients.* London: HMSO, 1989.
2 Gale T. *The Court of the Gentiles; or, a discourse touching the original of human literature, both philologic and philosophic, from the scriptures and Jewish Churches.* Oxford and London, 1667. Part III, Book I, Chap 4. p. 87.
3 Arnold M. *Essays in criticism.* London, 1865.
4 *Medical Audit.* Working paper 6 accompanying 'Working for patients'. London: HMSO, 1989.
5 *Medical audit: a first report.* London: Royal College of Physicians, 1989.
6 Shaw C. *Medical audit.* A hospital handbook. London: King's Fund Centre, 1989.
6a Stone DH. Proposed taxonomy of audit and related activities. *J R Coll Physicians Lond* 1990; **24**: 30–31.

7 Gospel according to St. Matthew 25: 19–30.

8 Brook RH, Kosecoff JB. Commentary: competition and quality. *Health Affairs*, 1988; **7**: 150–161.

9 Donabedian A. Evaluating the quality of medical care. *Millbank Memorial Fund Quarterly* 1966; **44: Suppl.** 166–206.

10 Donabedian A. *Needed research in the assessment and monitoring of the quality of medical care*. Washington: US Department of Health, Education and Welfare. National Center for Health Services Research, DHEW Publication No. (PHS) 78-3219, 1978.

11 Donabedian A. *Explorations in quality assessment and monitoring. 1. The definition of quality and approaches to its assessment*. Ann Arbor: Health Administration Press, 1980.

12 Donabedian A. *Explorations in quality assessment and monitoring. 2. The criteria and standards of quality*. Ann Arbor: Health Administration Press, 1982.

13 Donabedian A. *Explorations in quality assessment and monitoring. 3. The methods and findings of quality assessment and monitoring*. Ann Arbor: Health Administration Press, 1985.

14 Donabedian A. The quality of care. How can it be assessed? *J Am Med Assoc* 1989; **260**: 1743–1748.

15 McCance DR, Atkinson AB, Hadden DR *et al*. Longterm glycaemic control and diabetic retinopathy. *Lancet* 1989; **2**: 824–828.

16 Karjalainen S, Palva I. Do treatment protocols improve end results? A study of survival of patients with multiple myeloma in Finland. *Br Med J* 1989; **299**: 1069–1072.

17 Cochrane AL. *Effectiveness and efficiency: random reflections on health services*. London: Nuffield Provincial Hospitals Trust, 1972.

18 Chassin MR, Park RE, Fink A *et al*. *Indications for selected medical and surgical procedures — a literature review and ratings of appropriateness*. Coronary artery bypass graft surgery. Santa Monica: RAND Corporation. Publication No. - 3204/2-CWF/HF/HCFA/PMT/RWJ, 1986.

19 US Congress, Office of Technology Assessment. *The Quality of Medical Care: Information for Consumers*. Washington D.C. U.S. Government Printing Office. Publication No. OTA-H-386, 1988.

20 Kahn KL, Kosecoff J, Chassin MR *et al*. Measuring the clinical appropriateness of the use of a procedure: can we do it? *Med Care* 1988; **26**: 415–422.

21 King M. *Personal health care: the quest for a human right. Human rights in health*. Ciba Foundation Symposium 23 (new series). London: Ciba Foundation, 1974.

22 Maxwell RJ. Quality assessment in health. *Br Med J* 1984; **288**: 1470–1472.

23 Tarlov AR, Ware JE, Greenfield S *et al*. The Medical Outcomes Study: the application of methods for monitoring the results of medical care. *J Am Med Assoc* 1989; **262**: 925–930.

24 Editorial. Health care inequity in the USA. *Lancet* 1988; **2**: 316–317.

25 Fox J. Social network interaction: new jargon in health inequalities. *Br Med J* 1988; **297**: 373–374.

26 Eyles J, Woods K. Who cares what care? An inverse interest law? *Social Sci Med* 1986; **23**: 1087–1092.

27 Hewer RL, Wood VA. A report on neurology services in the United Kingdom. Bristol: Department of Neurology, Frenchay Hospital, 1988.

28 Garrison LP, Bowman MA, Perrin EB. Estimating physician requirements for neurology: a needs-based approach. *Neurology* 1984; **34**: 1218–1227.

29 Menken M, Hopkins A, Murray TJ, Vates TS. The scope of neurologic practice and care in England, Canada and the United States: is there is a better way? *Arch Neurol* 1989; **46**: 210–213.

30 Hopkins A. Auditing performance in clinical rheumatology. In: Scott DL, Baillie K, eds. *Measuring performance in clinical rheumatology*. London: The

Arthritis and Rheumatism Council for Research. Conference proceedings No. 7, 1990.

31 National Association of Health Authorities. *The nation's health: a way forward.* Birmingham: National Association of Health Authorities, 1988.

32 Black N. An inspector calls.' *Br Med J* 1988; **297**: 875.

33 Culyer AJ. *Competition and markets in health care: What we know and what we don't.* NHS White Paper. Occasional Paper 3. York: Centre for Health Economics, Health Economics Consortium, 1989.

34 Cherkin DC, Grothaus L, Wagner EH. The effect of office visit copayments on utilisation in a health care organisation. *Med Care* 1989; **27**: 669–679.

35 Epstein AM, Stern RS, Weissman JS. Do the poor cost more? A multihospital study of patients' socioeconomic status and use of hospital resources. *N Engl J Med* 1990; **322:** 1122–1128.

36 Hayward RA, Shapiro MF, Freeman HE, Corey CR. Inequities in health services among insured Americans. Do working-age adults have less access to medical care than the elderly? *N Engl J Med* 1988; **318**: 1507–1512.

37 Braveman P, Oliva G, Miller MG *et al.* Adverse outcomes and lack of health insurance among newborns in an eight-county area of California,1982–1986. *N Engl J Med* 1989; **321**: 508–513.

38 Coopers and Lybrand. *Report on Radiotherapy Services to the North East Thames Regional Health Authority.* London, 1987.

39 Yi J-j, Rowley JM, Hampton JR. The appropriate use of investigations in cardiology. In: Hopkins A, ed. *Appropriate investigation and treatment.* London: Royal College of Physicians, 1989.

40 Berwick DM. Quality assurance and measurement principles: the perspective from one health maintenance organisation. In: Hughes EFX, ed. *Perspectives on quality in American health care.* Washington, D.C.: McGraw-Hill, 1988.

41 Bulpitt CJ. Meta-analysis. *Lancet* 1988; **2**: 93–94.

42 Schwartz JS, Ball JR, Moser RH. Safety, efficacy, and the effectiveness of clinical practice. *Ann Intern Med* 1982; **96**: 246.

42a Brook RH. Practice guidelines and practicing medicine. Are they compatible? *J Am Med Assoc* 1982; **262**: 3027–3030.

42b Eddy DM. Clinical decision making: from theory to practice. Practice policies — what are they? *J Am Med Assoc* 1990; **263**: 877–880.

43 Consensus conference: treatment of stroke. *Br Med J* 1988; **297**: 126–128.

44 Lomas J, Anderson G, Enkin M *et al.* The role of evidence in the consensus process. *J Am Med Assoc* 1988; **259**: 3001–3005.

45 Lomas J, Anderson GM, Domnick-Pierre K *et al.* Do practice guidelines guide practice? The effect of a consensus statement on the practice of physicians. *N Engl J Med* 1989; **321**: 1306–1311.

46 Zeitlin GL. Possible decrease in mortality associated with anaesthesia. A comparison of two time periods in Massachusetts, USA. *Anaesthesia* 1989; **44**: 432–433.

47 Wennberg J, Gittelsohn A. Variations in medical care among small areas. *Scientific American* 1982; **246** (4): 120–135.

48 Chassin MR, Brook RH, Park RE. Variations in the use of medical and surgical services by the Medicare population. *N Engl J Med* 1986; **314**: 285–290.

49 Wennberg JE, Freeman JL, Culp WJ. Are hospital services rationed in New Haven or over-utilised in Boston? *Lancet* 1987; **1**: 1185–1189.

50 Perrin JM, Homer CJ, Berwick DM *et al.* Variations in rates of hospitalisation of children in three urban communities. *N Engl J Med* 1989; **320**: 1183–1187.

51 UK–TIA Study Group. Variation in the use of angiography and carotid endarterectomy by neurologists in the UK–TIA aspirin trial. *Br Med J* 1983; **286**: 514–517.

52 Wilkin D, Metcalfe DH, Marinker M. The meaning of information on GP refer-

ral rates to hospitals. *Community Med* 1989; **11**: 65–70.

53 Brook RH, Kosecoff JB, Park RE *et al.* Diagnosis and treatment of coronary disease: comparison of doctors attitudes in the USA and UK. *Lancet* 1988; **1**: 750–753.

54 Hopkins A, Menken M, DeFriese GH, Feldman AG. Differences in strategies for the diagnosis and treatment of neurological disease among British and American neurologists. *Arch Neurol* 1989; **46**: 1142–1148.

55 Kemper KJ. Medically inappropriate hospital use in a paediatric population. *N Engl J Med* 1988; **318**: 1033–1037.

56 Selker HP, Beshansky JR, Pauker SG, Kassirer JP. The epidemiology of delays in a teaching hospital. The development of a tool that detects unnecessary hospital days. *Med Care* 1989; **27**: 112–129.

57 Anderson P, Meara J, Broadhurst S *et al.* Use of hospital beds: a cohort study of admissions to a provincial teaching hospital. *Br Med J* 1988; **297**: 910–912.

58 Wennberg JE, Freeman JL, Shelton RM, Bubolz TA. Hospital use and mortality among Medicare beneficiaries in Boston and New Haven. *N Engl J Med* 1989; **321**: 1168–1173.

59 Hopkins A, Garman A, Clarke C. The first seizure in adult life: value of electro-encephalography and computerised scanning in prediction of seizure recurrence. *Lancet* 1988; **1**: 721–727.

60 Hopkins A. Appropriate investigation in neurology. In: Hopkins A, ed. *Appropriate use of investigation and treatment in clinical practice.* London: Royal College of Physicians, 1989.

60a Leape LL, Park RE, Solomon DH *et al.* Does inappropriate use explain small-area variations in the use of health care services? *J Am Med Assoc* 1990; **263**: 669–672.

61 Wald NJ. Rational use of investigations in clinical practice. In: Hopkins A, ed. *Appropriate investigation and treatment in clinical practice.* London: Royal College of Physicians, 1989.

62 Weinstein MC, Fineberg HV. *Clinical decision analysis.* Philadelphia: WB Saunders, 1985.

63 Dowie J, Elstein AS. *Professional judgement: a reader in clinical decision making.* New York: Cambridge University Press, 1988.

64 Balla JI, Elstein AS, Chistiansen C. Obstacles to acceptance of clinical decision analysis. *Br Med J* 1989; **298**: 579–582.

65 Eddy DM. Success and challenges of medical decision making. *Health Affairs* 1986; Summer, 1986: 108–115.

66 Howard RA. Microrisks for medical decision analysis. *Int J Technol Assess Hlth Care* 1989; **5**: 357–370.

67 Hellinger FJ. Expected utility theory and risky choices with health outcomes. *Med Care* 1989; **27**: 273–279.

68 *Clinical algorithms: central nervous system; gynaecology; endocrine system.* London: British Medical Journal Publications, 1989.

68a Flanagin A, Lundberg GD. Clinical decision making: promoting the jump from theory to practice. *J Am Med Assoc* 1990; **263**: 279–280.

68b Eddy DM. Clinical decision making: from theory to practice. The challenge. *J Am Med Assoc* 1990; **263**: 287–290.

68c Hopkins A, Scambler G. How doctors deal with epilepsy. *Lancet* 1977; **2**: 183–186.

69 Fletcher CM. *Communication in medicine.* London: Nuffield Provincial Hospitals Trust, 1973.

70 Bourhis RY, Roth S, MacQueen G. Communication in the hospital setting: a survey of medical and everyday language use amongst patients, nurses and doctors. *Social Sci Med* 1989; **28**: 339–346.

71 Tattersall RB. Informing patients. *Lancet* 1989; **2**: 280.

72 Quill TE. Recognising and adjusting to barriers in doctor–patient communication. *Ann Intern Med* 1989; **111**: 51–57.

73 Harrigan JA, Gramata JF, Lucic KS, Margolis C. It's how you say it: physicians' vocal behaviour. *Social Sci Med* 1989; **28**: 87–92.

74 *Annual Report of Massachusetts Peer Review Organisation*. Boston: MassPRO, 1989.

75 Heath D. Random review of hospital patient records. *Brit Med J* 1990; **300**: 651–652.

76 Feldstein PJ, Wickizer TM, Wheeler JRC. Private cost containment. The effects of utilisation review programs in health care use and expenditure. *N Engl J Med* 1988; **318**: 1310–1314.

77 Empire Blue Cross and Blue Shield. *How to comply with Empire Blue Cross and Blue Shield Managed Care*. Empire Blue Cross and Blue Shield; New York, 1988.

78 Wickizer TM, Wheeler JRC, Feldstein PJ. Does utilisation review reduce unnecessary hospital care and contain costs? *Med Care* 1989; **27**: 632–647.

79 Rosenberg SN, Gorman SA, Snitzer S, Herbst EV, Lynne D. Patients' reactions and physician patient communication in a mandatory surgical second opinion program. *Med Care* 1989; **27**: 466–477.

80 Kosecoff J. Personal communication, 1989.

81 Rutstein DD, Berenberg W, Chalmers TC *et al*. Measuring the quality of medical care: second revision of tables of indexes. *N Engl J Med* 1980; **302**: 1146, 294, 582–588.

82 Charlton JRH, Silver RM, Hartley RM *et al*. Geographical variation in mortality from conditions amenable to medical intervention in England and Wales. *Lancet* 1983; **1**: 691–696.

83 Charlton JRH, Bauer RL, Lakhani AZ. Outcome measures for district and regional planner. *Community Med* 1984; **6**: 306–315.

84 Mackenbach JP, Stronks K, Kunst AE. The contribution of medical care to inequalities in health: differences between socio-economic groups in decline of mortality from conditions amenable to medical intervention. *Social Sci Med* 1989; **29**: 369–376.

85 US Congress, Office of Technology Assessment. *The quality of medical care: information for consumers*. OTA-H-386. Washington, DC: US Government Printing Office.

86 Fink A, Yano EM, Brook RH. The condition of the literature on differences in hospital mortality. *Med Care* 1989; **27**: 315–335.

87 Iezzoni LI. Measuring the severity of illness and case-mix. In: Goldfield N, Nash DB, eds. *Providing quality care*. Philadelphia: Am Coll Physicians, 1989.

88 Knaus WA, Draper EA, Wagner DP, Zimmerman JE. APACHE II: a severity of disease classification system. *Crit Care Med* 1985; **13**: 818–829.

89 Knaus WA, Draper EA, Wagner DP, Zimmerman JE. An evaluation of outcome from intensive care in major centres. *Ann Intern Med* 1986; **104**: 410–418.

90 Tarnow-Mordi W, Ogston S, Wilkinson AR *et al*. Predicting death from initial disease severity in very low birth weight infants: a method for comparing the performance of neonatal units. *Brit Med J* (in press).

91 Pollack MM, Ruttimann UE, Getson PR *et al*. Accurate prediction of the outcome of paediatric intensive care. *N Engl J Med* 1987; **316**: 134–139.

92 Health Care Financing Administration. *Medicare hospital mortality information*. GPO publication no. 1987 0-1968 60. Washington DC: Government Printing Office, 1968.

93 Berwick DM. Continuous improvement as an ideal in health care. *N Engl J Med* 1989; **320**: 53–56.

93a Green J, Wintfield N, Sharkey P, Passman LJ. The importance of severity of illness in assessing hospital mortality. *J Am Med Assoc* 1990; **263**: 241–246.

94 Dubois RW, Rogers WH, Moxley JH *et al*. Hospital inpatient mortality. Is it a predictor of quality? *N Engl J Med* 1987; **317**: 1674–1680.

94a Hartz AJ, Krakauer H, Kuhn EM *et al.* Hospital characteristics and mortality rates. *N Engl J Med* 1989; **321**: 1720–1725.

95 Dubois RW, Brook RH. Preventable deaths: who, how often, and why? *Ann Intern Med* 1988; **109**: 582–589.

96 Buck N, Devlin HB, Lunn JN. *The report of a confidential enquiry into perioperative deaths.* London: Nuffield Provincial Hospitals Trust and The King's Fund, 1988.

97 Mugford M, Kingston J, Chalmers I. Reducing the incidence of infection after Caesarean section: implications of prophylaxis with antibiotics for hospital resources. *Br Med J* 1989; **299**: 1003–1006.

98 Silberstein LE, Kruskall MS, Stehling LC *et al.* Strategies for the review of transfusion practices. *J Am Med Assoc* 1989; **262**: 1993–1997.

99 Henderson J, Goldacre MJ, Graveney MJ, Simmons HM. Use of medical record linkage to study readmission rates. *Br Med J* 1989; **299**: 709–713.

99a Gold BS, Kitz DS, Lecky JH, Neuhaus JM. Unanticipated admission to the hospital following day case surgery. *J Am Med Assoc* 1989; **262**: 3008–3010.

100 Nevitt MC, Cummings SR, Kidd S, Black D. Risk factors for recurrent non-surgical falls: a prospective study. *J Am Med Assoc* 1989; **261**: 2663–2668.

101 Morse JM, Black C, Oberle K, Donahue P. A prospective study to identify the fall-prone patient. *Social Sci Med* 1989; **28**: 81–86.

102 Leape LL, Park RE, Soloman DH *et al.* Relation between surgeons' practice volumes and geographic variations in the rate of carotid endarterectomy. *N Engl J Med* 1989; **321**: 653–657.

103 Hannan EL, O'Donnell JF, Kilburn H. Bernard HR, Yazici A. Investigation of the relationship between volume and mortality for surgical procedures performed in New York State hospitals. *J Am Med Assoc* 1989; **262**: 503–510.

104 Gruer R, Gunn AA, Gordon DS, Ruckley CV. Audit of surgical audit. *Lancet* 1986; **1**: 23–26.

105 Codman EA. The product of a hospital. *Surg Gynaec Obstet* 1914; **18**: 491–496.

106 Bennett CL, Garfinkle JB, Greenfield S *et al.* The relationship between hospital experience and in hospital mortality for patients with AIDS-related PCP. *J Am Med Assoc* 1989; **261**: 2975–2979.

107 Rawson MD, Liversedge LA. Treatment of retrobulbar neuritis with corticotrophin. *Lancet* 1969; **2**: 222.

108 Kaplan RM, Atkins CJ, Timms R. Validity of a quality of well-being scale as an outcome measure in chronic obstructive pulmonary disease. *J Chron Dis* 1984; **37**: 85–95.

109 Tattersfield A. Personal communication.

110 Bull BS, Farr M, Meyer PJ *et al.* Efficacy of tests used to monitor rheumatoid arthritis. *Lancet* 1989; **2**: 965–967.

111 Wells KB, Stewart A, Hays RD *et al.* The functioning and well-being of depressed patients: results from the Medical Outcomes Study. *J Am Med Assoc* 1989; **262**: 914–919.

112 Henderson RA, Bucknall CA, Timmis AD *et al.* Clinical outcome of coronary angioplasty for single-vessel disease. *Lancet* 1989; **2**: 546–550.

113 Ware JE. Standards for validating health measures: definition and content. *J Chron Dis* 1987; **40**: 473–480.

114 Segovia J, Bartlett RF, Edwards AC. An empirical analysis of the dimensions of health status measures. *Social Sci Med* 1989; **29**: 761–768.

115 O'Brien BJ, Banner NR, Gibson S, Yacoub MH. The Nottingham Health Profile as a measure of quality of life following combined heart and lung transplantation. *J Epidemiol Comm Hlth* 1988; **42**: 232–234.

116 Selby PJ, Chapman JAW, Etzadi-Amoli *et al.* The development of a method for assessing the quality of life of cancer patients. *Br J Cancer* 1984; **50**: 13–22.

116a Evans RW, Rader B, Manninen DL and the Cooperative Multicenter EPO

Clinical Trial Group. The quality of life of hemodialysis recipients treated with recombinant human erythropoietin. *J Am Med Assoc* 1990; **263**: 825–830.

117 Ebbs SR, Fallowfield LJ, Fraser SCA, Baum M. Treatment outcomes and quality of life. *Int J Technol Assess Hlth Care* 1989; **5**: 391–400.

118 Slevin ML, Plant H, Lynch D *et al.* Who should measure the quality of life, the doctor or the patient? *Br J Cancer* 1988; **57**: 109–112.

119 Kind P. *The design and construction of quality of life measures.* Discussion Paper 43. Centre for Health Economics. York: Centre for Health Economics, (undated).

120 Teeling-Smith G, ed. *Measuring health: a practical approach.* Chichester etc: John Wiley and Sons, 1988.

121 Advances in health status assessment. *Med Care* 1989; **27**: **Suppl** S1-S294.

122 Mahoney FI, Barthel DW. Functional evaluation: the Barthel index. *Maryland State Med J* 1965; **14**: 61–65.

123 Ebrahim S, Nouri F, Barer D. Measuring disability after a stroke. *J Epidemiol Comm Hlth* 1985; **39**: 86–89.

124 Stewart AL, Hays RD, Ware JE. The MOS short-form general health survey: reliability and validity in a patient population. *Med Care* 1988; **26**: 724–735.

125 Stewart AL, Greenfield S, Wells K *et al.* Functional status and well-being of patients with chronic conditions: results from the Medical Outcomes Study. *J Am Med Assoc* 1989; **262**: 907–913.

126 Croog SH, Levine S, Testa MA *et al.* The effects of antihypertensive therapy on the quality of life. *N Engl J Med* 1986; **314**: 1657–1664.

127 Torrance GW. Utility approach to measuring health-related quality of life. *J Chron Dis* 1987; **40**: 593–600.

127a Torrance GW, Feeny D. Utilities and quality-adjusted life years. *Int J Technol Assess Hlth Care* 1989; **5**: 559–575.

128 Buxton M, Ashby S. The time trade-off approach to health state valuation. In: Teeling-Smith G, ed. *Measuring health: a practical approach.* Chichester etc: John Wiley and Sons, 1988.

129 Capewell G. Techniques of health status measurement using a health index. In: Teeling-Smith G ed. *Measuring health: a practical approach.* Chichester etc: John Wiley and Sons, 1988.

130 Rosser RM, Watts VC. The measurement of hospital output. *Int J Epidemiol* 1972; **1**: 361–368.

131 Rosser RM. From health indicators to quality adjusted life-years: technical and ethical issues. In: Hopkins A, Costain D, eds. *Measuring the outcomes of medical care.* London: Royal College of Physicians, 1990

132 Williams A. The economic evaluation of coronary bypass grafts. *Br Med J* 1985; **291**: 326–329.

133 Fries JF, Green LW, Levine S. Health promotion and the compression of morbidity. *Lancet* 1989; **1**: 481–483.

134 Leaf A. Cost effectiveness as a criteria for Medicare coverage. *N Engl J Med* 1989; **321**: 898–900.

135 Weinstein MC, Stason WB. Foundations of cost-effectiveness analysis for health and medical practices. *N Engl J Med* 1977; **296**: 716–721.

136 Klein R. The role of health economics. *Br Med J* 1989; **299**: 275–276.

137 Morris JN. Suissa S, Sherwood S *et al.* Last days: a study of terminally ill cancer patients. *J Chron Dis* 1986; **39**: 47–62.

138 Nelson EC, Berwick DM. The measurement of health status in clinical practice. *Med Care* 1989; **27**: **Suppl.** S77–S90.

139 Ebrahim S. Measurement of impairment, disability and handicap. In: Hopkins A, Costain D, eds. *Measuring the outcomes of medical care.* London: Royal College of Physicians, 1990.

140 Williams TF, Hill JG, Fairbank MF *et al.* Appropriate placement of the chronically ill and aged: a successful approach by evaluation. *J Am Med Assoc* 1973; **226**: 1332–1335.

141 Lewis MA, Leake B, Clark V, Leal-Sotelo M. Case mix and outcomes of nursing home patients: the importance of prior nursing home care, and admission from home versus hospital. *Med Care* 1989; **27**: 376–385.

142 Spiegel D, Kraemer HC, Bloom JR, Gothheil E. Effect of psychosocial treatment on survival of patients with metastatic breast cancer. *Lancet* 1989; **2**: 889–891.

143 Siegrist J. Impaired quality of life as a risk factor in cardiovascular disease. *J Chron Dis* 1987; **40**: 571–578.

144 Gibson RM, Stephenson GC. Aggressive management of severe closed head trauma: time for re-appraisal. *Lancet* 1989; **2**: 369–370.

145 Nevitt MP, Ballard DJ, Hallet JW. Prognosis of abdominal aortic aneurysms: a population based study. *N Engl J Med* 1989; **321**: 1009–1014.

146 Greenfield S. The state of outcome research: are we on target? *N Engl J Med* 1989; **320**: 1142–1143.

147 Drummond MF. Resource allocation decisions in health care: a role for quality of life assessments? *J Chron Dis* 1987; **40**: 605–616.

148 Eisenberg JM. Clinical economics. *J Am Med Assoc* 1989; **262**: 2879–2886.

149 Welch HG. Health care tickets for the uninsured: first class, coach or standby. *N Engl J Med* 1989; **321**: 1261–1264.

150 MRC Working Party. MRC trial of treatment of mild hypertension: principal results. *Br Med J* 1985; **291**: 97–104.

151 Wilcox RG, Mitchell JRA, Hampton JR. Treatment of high blood pressure: should clinical practice be based on results of clinical trials? *Br Med J* 1986; **293**: 433–437.

152 Laupacis A, Sackett DL, Roberts RS. An assessment of clinically useful measures of the consequences of treatment. *N Engl J Med* 1988; **318**: 1728–1733.

153 Vladeck BC. Hospital prospective payment and quality of care. *N Engl J Med* 1988; **319**: 1411–1413.

154 Schramm CJ, Gabel J. Prospective payment: some retrospective observations. *N Engl J Med* 1988; **318**: 1681–1683.

155 Fitzgerald JF, Moore PS, Dittus RS. The care of elderly patients with hip fracture: changes since implementation of the prospective payment system. *N Engl J Med* 1988; **319**: 1392–1397.

156 Sager MA, Easterling DV, Kindig DA, Anderson OW. Changes in the location of death after passage of Medicare's prospective payment system: a national study. *N Engl J Med* 1989; **320**: 433–439.

157 Hopkins A, Maxwell R. Contracts and quality of care. *Br Med J* 1990; **300**: 919–922.

158 Cleary PD, McNeil BJ. Patient satisfaction as an indicator of quality of care. *Inquiry* 1988; **25**: 25–36.

159 Department of Health and Social Security. *Health Service Management. Hospital Complaints Procedure Act 1985.* Health Circular HC(88)37 HN(FP)(88)18. London: Department of Health and Social Security, 1988.

160 Sunol R, Delgado R, Pacheco MV, Baures N. *Methods to evaluate patient satisfaction.* Proceedings of an international symposium on quality assurance. Shanahan M, ed. Chicago, Illinois: Joint Commission on Accreditation of Hospitals, 1987.

161 Jones L, Leneman L, Maclean U. *Consumer feedback for the NHS: a literature review.* London: King Edward's Hospital Fund for London, 1987.

162 Cryns AG, Nichols RC, Katz LA, Calkins E. The hierarchical structure of geriatric patient satisfaction. An older patient satisfaction scale designed for HMOS. *Med Care* 1989; **27**: 802–816.

163 Ware JE, Snyder MK, Wright WR, Davies AR. Defining and measuring patient satisfaction with medical care. *Evaluation and Program Planning* 1983; **6**: 247–263.
164 Fitzpatrick R. The measurement of satisfaction. In: Hopkins A, Costain D, eds. *Measuring the outcomes of medical care.* London: Royal College of Physicians (in press).
165 Stiles W, Putnam S, Wolf M, James S. Interaction exchange structure and patient satisfaction with medical interviews. *Med Care* 1979; **17**: 667–679.
166 Crown J, Harvey J, Kerruish A, Wickings I. Proof of the pudding. *Health Service J* 1989; **99**: 1070–1071.
167 Carr-Hill R, Dixon P, Thompson A. Too simple for words. *Health Service J* 1989; **99**: 728–729.
168 Carr-Hill R, Dixon P, Thompson A. Putting patients before the machine. *Health Service J* 1989; **99**: 1132–1133.
169 Fitzpatrick M, Hopkins A. Referrals to neurologists for headaches not due to structural disease. *J Neurol Neurosurg Psychiat* 1981; **44**: 1061–1067.
170 Thompson A. Patient satisfaction and the quality of care. *Int J Qual Assurance* (in press).
171 Davies AR, Ware JE. Involving consumers in quality of care assessment. *Health Affairs* 1988; **7**: 33–48.
172 Sox HC, Margulies I, Sox CM. Psychologically mediated effects of diagnostic tests. *Ann Intern Med* 1981; **95**: 680–685.
173 Rashid A, Forman W, Jagger C, Mann R. Consultations in general practice: a comparison of patients' and doctors' satisfaction. *Br Med J* 1989; **299**: 1015–1016.
174 Sunol R. Doctoral thesis: University of Barcelona, 1989.
175 Thompson A. *The measurement of patients' perceptions of the quality of hospital care.* Doctoral thesis: University of Manchester, 1983.
176 Marteau TM. Psychological costs of screening. *Br Med J* 1989; **299**: 527.
177 Oboler SK, Laforce FM. The periodic physical examination in asymptomatic adults. *Ann Intern Med* 1989; **110**: 214–226.
178 Eddy DM. Screening for lung cancer. *Ann Intern Med* 1989; **111**: 232–237.
179 Holland WW, Stewart S. *Screening in health care — benefit or bane?* London: Nuffield Provincial Hospitals Trust,1990.
180 Warner KE, Wickizer TM, Wolfre RA *et al.* Economic implications of work place health promotion programs: review of the literature. *J Occupat Med* 1988; **30**: 106–112.
181 Editorial. Health promotion at work. *Lancet* 1988; **2**: 832.
182 Engleman S. The impact of mass media anti-smoking publicity. *Health Promotion* 1987; **2**: 63–74.
183 Smith CH, Armstrong D. Comparison of criteria derived by government and patients for evaluating general practitioner services. *Br Med J* 1989; **299**: 494–496.
184 Emerson PA, Russell NJ, Wyatt J *et al.* An audit of doctors' management of patients with chest pain in the accident and emergency department. *Q J Med* 1989; **NS 70**: 213–220.
185 Sharkey SW, Brunette DD, Ruiz E *et al.* An analysis of time delays preceding thrombolysis for acute myocardial infarction. *J Am Med Assoc* 1989; **262**: 3171–3174.
186 Winner S, Boon N. Clinical problems with temporary pacemakers prior to permanent pacing. *J R Coll Physicians Lond* 1989; **23**: 161–163.
186a Gentleman D, Jennett B. Audit of transfer of unconscious head-injured patients to a neurosurgical unit. *Lancet* 1990; **335**: 330–334.
186b Reeve WG, Runcie CJ, Reidy J, Wallace PGM. Current practice in transferring critically ill patients among hospitals in the West of Scotland. *Br Med J* 1990; **300**: 85–87.

187 Morrisey S, Alun-Jones T, Leighton S. Why are operations cancelled? *Br Med J* 1989; **299**: 778.

188 Rooks JP, Weatherby NL, Ernst EKM *et al.* Outcomes of care in birth centers. *N Engl J Med* 1989; **321**: 1804–1811.

189 Black PC, Ockene I, Goldberg RJ *et al.* A prospective randomised trial of out-patient versus inpatient catheterisation. *N Engl J Med* 1988; **319**: 1251–1255.

189a Petty R, Gumpel M. Acute medical admissions: changes following a sudden reduction in bed numbers at Northwick Park Hospital. *J R Coll Physicians Lond* 1990; **24**: 32–35.

189b Howarth S, Clarke C, Bayliss R *et al.* Mortality in elderly patients admitted for respite care. *Br Med J* 1990; **300**: 844–847.

190 Howie JGR, Porter AMD, Forbes JF. Quality and the use of time in general practice: widening the discussion. *Br Med J* 1989; **298**: 1008–1010.

191 Palmer FB, Shapiro BK, Wachtel RC *et al.* The effects of physical therapy on cerebral palsy: a controlled trial in infants with spastic diplegia. *N Engl J Med* 1988; **318**: 803–808.

192 McKinney LA. Early mobilisation and outcome in acute sprains of the neck. *Br Med J* 1989; **299**: 1006–1008.

193 Costigan PS, Miller G, Elliott C, Wallace WA. Are surgical shoes providing value for money? *Br Med J* 1989; **299**: 950.

194 Masters SJ, McLean PM, Arcarese JS *et al.* Skull X-ray after trauma. Recommendations by a multidisciplinary panel and validation study. *N Engl J Med* 1987; **316**: 84–91.

195 Page JE, Olliff JFC, Dundas DD. Value of anterior-posterior radiography in cervical pain of non-traumatic origin. *Br Med J* 1989; **298**: 1293–1294.

196 Heller CA, Stanley P, Lewis-Jones B, Heller RF. Value of X-ray examinations of the cervical spine. *Br Med J* 1983; **287**: 1274–1278.

197 Hubbell FA, Greenfield S, Tyler JL *et al.* The impact of routine chest X-ray films on patient care. *N Engl J Med* 1985; **312**: 209–213.

198 Sandercock PAG, Roberts MA, Blumhardt LD. A prospective audit of the use and costs of myelography in a regional neuroscience unit. *J Neurol Neurosurg Psychiat* 1989; **52**: 1078–1084.

199 Bransby-Zachary MAP, Sutherland GR. Unnecessary X-ray examinations. *Br Med J* 1989; **298**: 1294.

199a Vallely SR, Mills JOM. Should radiologists talk to patients? *Br Med J* 1990; **300**: 305–306.

200 Morgan AG. Is routine urine testing in outpatient clinics useful? *Br Med J* 1988; **297**: 1173.

201 Campbell IT, Gosling P. Preoperative biochemical screening. *Br Med J* 1988; **297**: 803.

201a Routine diagnostic testing. *Lancet* 1989; **2**: 1190–1191.

202 Flanagan PG, Rooney PG, Davies EA, Stout RW. Evaluation of four screening tests for bacteriuria in elderly people. *Lancet* 1989; **1**: 1117–1119.

203 McCance DC, Hadden DR, Atkinson AB, Archer DB, Kennedy L. Long term glycaemic control and diabetic retinopathy. *Lancet* 1989; **2**: 824–827.

203a Patchall RA, Tibbs PA, Walsh JW *et al.* A randomized trial of surgery in the treatment of single metastasis to the brain. *N Engl J Med* 1990; **322**: 494–500.

203b Evans GR, Taylor G, Taylor KG. The work of a lipid clinic: an audit of performance. *Q J Med* 1990; **NS 74**: 239–245.

204 Raju TNK, Kecskes S, Thornton JP, Perry M, Feldman S. Medication errors in neonatal and paediatric intensive care units. *Lancet* 1989; **2**: 374–376.

204a Beers MH, Storrie M, Lee G. Potential adverse drug interactions in the emergency room. *Ann Intern Med* 1990; **112**: 61–64.

204b Shaw CD, Costain DW. Guidelines for medical audit: seven principles. *Br Med J* 1989; **299**: 498–499.

204c Weed LL. *Medical records, medical education and patient care.* Ohio: Press of Case

Western Reserve University, 1971.

205 Wiener CL, Kayer-Jones J. Defensive work in nursing homes: accountability gone amok. *Social Sci Med* 1989; **28**: 37–44.

206 Grumet GW. Health care rationing through inconvenience: the third party's secret weapon. *N Engl J Med* 1989; **321**: 607–611.

207 Roper WL, Winkenwerder W, Hackbarth GM, Krakauer H. Effectiveness in health care: an initiative to evaluate and improve medical practice. *N Engl J Med* 1988; **319**: 1197–1202.

208 Editorial. Databases for health care outcomes. *Lancet* 1989; **2**: 195–196.

209 Roos NP, Wennberg JE, Malenka DJ *et al.* Mortality and reoperation after open and transurethral resection of the prostate for benign prostatic hyperplasia. *N Engl J Med* 1989; **320**: 1120–1124.

210 Coles C. Self assessment and medical audit: an educational approach. *Br Med J* 1989; **299**: 807–808.

211 Ellwood PM. Outcomes management: a technology of patient experience. *N Engl J Med* 1988; **318**: 1549–1556.

212 Brook RH. Practice guidelines and practising medicine: are they compatible? *J Am Med Assoc* 1989; **262**: 3027–3030.

213 Fowler FJ, Wennberg JE, Timothy RP *et al.* Symptom status and quality of life following prostatectomy. *J Am Med Assoc* 1988; **259**: 3018–3022.

214 Barry MJ, Mulley AG, Fowler FJ, Wennberg JW. Watchful waiting vs. immediate transurethral resection for symptomatic prostatism. The importance of patient preferences. *J Am Med Assoc* 1988; **259**: 3010–3017.

215 Loomes G, McKenzie L. The use of QALYs in health care decision making. *Social Sci Med* 1989; **28**: 299–308.

216 Carr-Hill RA. The evaluation of health care. *Social Sci Med* 1985; **21**: 367–375.

217 Rogers TF. Improving the fit between social science and health care practice: suggested next steps for the researcher. *Social Sci Med* 1987; **25**: 689–696.

218 Mitchell MW, Fowkes FGR. Audit reviewed: does feedback on performance change clinical behaviour? *J R Coll Physicians Lond* 1985; **19**: 251–254.

219 Eisenberg JM. *Doctors, decisions and the cost of medical care.* Ann Arbor: Health Administration Press, 1986.

220 Myers SA, Gleicher N. A successful program to lower Caesarian section rates. *N Engl J Med* 1988; **319**: 1511–1516.

220a Stafford RS. Alternative strategies for controlling rising Caesarean section rates. *J Am Med Assoc* 1990; **263**: 683–687.

221 Fowkes FGR. *Strategies for changing the use of diagnostic radiology.* Project Paper No. 57. London: King's Fund, 1986.

221a Manheim LM, Feinglass J, Hughes R *et al.* Training house officers to be cost conscious. Effects of an educational intervention on charges and length of stay. *Med Care* 1990; **28**: 29–42.

222 Relman AS. The National Leadership Commission's Health Care Plan. *N Engl J Med* 1989; **320**: 314–315.

223 Relman AS. Assessment and accountability: the third revolution. *N Engl J Med* 1988; **319**: 1220–1222.

224 Sullivan LW. The health care priorities of the Bush administration. *N Engl J Med* 1989; **321**: 125–128.

225 Laffel G, Blumenthal D. The case for using industrial management quality science in health care organisations. *J Am Med Assoc* 1989; **262**: 2869–2873.

226 Scholtes PR. *The team handbook: how to use teams to improve quality.* Madison, Wisconsin: Joiner Associates, 1988.

227 Hunt LM, Jordan B, Irwin S. Views of what's wrong: diagnosis and patients' concepts of illness. *Social Sci Med* 1989; **28**: 945–956.